CW00555917

Aromatherapy

A practical introduction

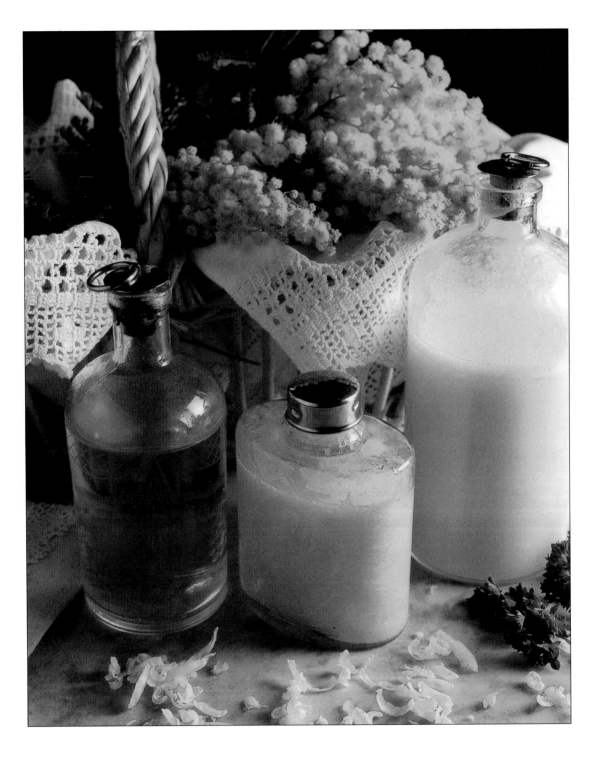

Aromatherapy

A practical introduction

Sandra White

Quantum
Books

A QUANTUM BOOK

This book is produced by
Quantum Publishing Ltd.
6 Blundell Street
London N7 9BH

Copyright ©MCMXCIX
Quantum Publishing Limited

This edition printed 2004

All rights reserved.
This book is protected by copyright. No part of it may be reproduced,
stored in a retrieval system, or transmitted in any form or by any means,
without the prior permission in writing of the Publisher, nor be otherwise
circulated in any form of binding or cover other than that in which it is
published and without a similar condition including this condition being
imposed on the subsequent publisher.

ISBN 1-86160-860-8

QUMAIA

Printed in Singapore by
Star Standard Industries Pte Ltd

This book is not intended as a substitute for the advice of a health care
professional. If you have any reason to believe you have a condition
which affects your health, you must seek professional advice. Consult a
qualified massage therapist, health care professional, aromatherapist or
your doctor before starting.

contents

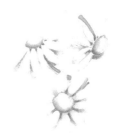

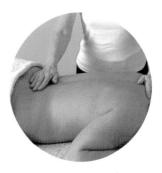

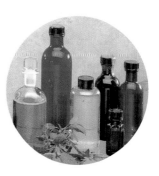

introduction to
Aromatherapy

The aim of this book is to introduce you to the fragrant world of 'Aromatherapy' a word which derives from 'aroma', meaning fragrance or smell and 'therapy' meaning treatment. This ancient healing art combines the aromatic essence of plants, known as essential oils, with relaxing massage.

A versatile holistic treatment, Aromatherapy is based on the ancient principle that the spirit and the body should be in harmony. By using a subtle combination of different essential oils, aromatherapy promotes both physical health, and mental and emotional well-being.

This book is intended to provide an introduction to the main essential oils, and to promote an understanding of how they are extracted, stored and used. A useful directory provides vital information on the properties of each oil, together with guidelines for safe usage, and effects and contra-indications to be aware of. The other key element of aromatherapy – massage – is then discussed, with basic massage strokes and techniques fully explained and demonstrated.

A full Aromatherapy treatment is a truly wonderful experience, combining, as it does, the beneficial properties of the essential oils with the warm relaxing atmosphere of a well prepared massage and possibly the enjoyment of soothing music which can appeal to the whole 'Mind, Body and Spirit'. However, this is not the only way that Aromatherapy can find a place in our busy lives. From fragrant baths to scented candles or oil burners, it can and does benefit and improve our day to day attitude to living.

Although it is one of the most ancient of the healing arts, Aromatherapy has only really become widely popular in the last few years. This increased popularity is largely due to people's growing awareness of the advantages of following a 'natural' path to health and fitness, rather than relying on conventional medicine. The effects of this new awareness can be felt in all areas

Making your own aromatherapy blends can be very satisfying

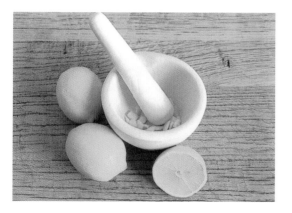

Oils can be extracted from many different parts of the plant or fruit.

of our lives today. More and more people have changed their diets as new information has become available regarding the benefits of fresh, natural foods, rather than the convenience or 'junk' foods favoured until recently. At the same time there has been growing appreciation and respect for what have often been termed as 'alternative' therapies, but which are more accurately described as 'complementary' therapies. These are the ancient and traditional treatments and remedies such as Aromatherapy and Reflexology that are now widely accepted as a complement to modern medicine, rather than as a replacement. By combining what is best from both the ancient healing arts and modern technology, we can truly achieve a healthy balance in both our physical and emotional lives.

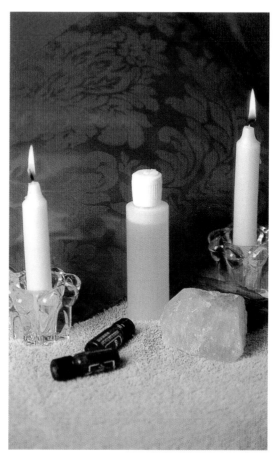

Creating a relaxing atmosphere is an essential part of aromatherapy

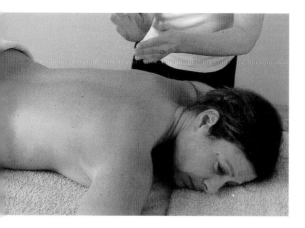

Aromatherapy combines the healing properties of essential oils with a relaxing massage.

IMPORTANT NOTICE

This book must not be used as a substitute for treatment of medical conditions when it is important that the help of a doctor is sought. The information is not intended to diagnose or treat and any safety guidelines covered throughout the book must be adhered to.

It is of particular importance that essential oils are not to be taken internally and all other contra-indications regarding the oils are closely observed.

history of Aromatherapy

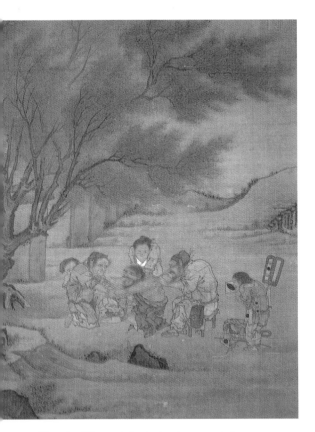

The ancient Chinese are believed to have been among the first practitioners of herbal medicine.

Aromatherapy is reputed to be at least 6000 years old, and is believed to have been practised by most of the world's ancient civilisations. Early man lived closely with his surroundings and was in tune with nature. His sense of smell was highly acute and herbs and aromatics were commonly used in the preservation of food, as aids to digestion or to treat a variety of ailments.

It is widely accepted that the Aromatherapy we know today can trace its origins back to ancient Egypt. A medical papyri believed to date back to around 1555 BC contains remedies for all types of illnesses, and many of the methods of application described are similar to those used in Aromatherapy and herbal medicine today.

The Egyptians used a method known as infusion (this process is described in a later chapter) to extract the oils from aromatic plants. One of the earliest ways of using aromatics was probably in the form of incense. For example, frankincense was commonly burned at sun rise as an offering to the sun god, Ra, while myrrh was offered to the moon. The Egyptians were also experts at embalming, and used aromatics to help preserve flesh. Yet aromatics had their place in pleasurable practices also, as the Egyptians enjoyed being massaged with fragrant oils after bathing.

There is evidence that the ancient Chinese civilisations were using some form of aromatics at a similar time to the Egyptians. Shen Nung's herbal book is the oldest surviving medical reference in China and dates back to around 2700 BC. This book contains information about over 300 plants. Like the Egyptians, the ancient Chinese also used aromatics in religious ceremonies, by burning aromatic woods and incense to show respect to their Gods. Their practice of using aromatics was linked to the equally ancient therapies of massage and acupressure.

Aromatherapy of some kind has also been in use for many centuries in India. The traditional Indian medicine, known as Ayurveda, has been practised for over 3000 years and this too, incorporates aromatic massage and the use of dried and fresh herbs as important aspects of the treatment.

The Greeks continued the practice of using aromatic oils begun by the Egyptians, and used them both medicinally and cosmetically. A Greek physician, Pedacius Dioscorides, wrote a definitive book about herbal medicine, and for at least 1200 years this was used as the Western world's standard medical reference. Many of the remedies he describes are still in use today.

The Romans took much of their medical knowledge from the Greeks, and they went on to refine and improve the use of aromatics, to the extent that Rome eventually became known as the bathing capital of the world. The popularity of scented baths followed by massage with aromatic oils is well documented, with public bath houses taking prominent positions in most towns. The popularity of aromatics lead to the opening up of extensive trading routes which enabled the Romans to import 'exotic' oils and spices from such far-away places as India and Arabia.

As the glory of the Roman Empire faded, the use of aromatics declined, with the knowledge of their use eventually being lost throughout Europe during the so-called dark ages. However, herbal and aromatic skills were still practised by some. One of the few places where the use of herbal medicine continued was in the monasteries, where the monks used plants from their herbal gardens to produce infused oils, herbal teas and medicines.

During the Middle Ages and the time of the plague, it was realised that certain aromatic substances seemed to help prevent the spread of infection, and aromatic woods such as cedar and pine were burnt to fumigate homes and streets.

The modern revival of the use of essential oils is thought to be due to a Persian physician and philosopher known as Avicenna who lived from AD 980 to AD 1037.

The Arabs began to use a method of distillation, and study of the therapeutic use of plants became popular in their Universities. During the Crusades this knowledge of distillation spread to the invading forces, and the lost process was brought back to Europe once more. By 1200 AD, essential oils were being produced in Germany, based mainly on herbs and spices brought from the Far East and Africa.

The invasions of South America by the conquistadors brought about the discovery of more medicinal plants and aromatic oils as the Spanish discovered the wealth of plant lore and remedies that had been used by the Aztecs for many centuries. Indeed, the vast range of medicinal plants found in Montezuma's botanical gardens formed the basis of many new and important remedies and treatments.

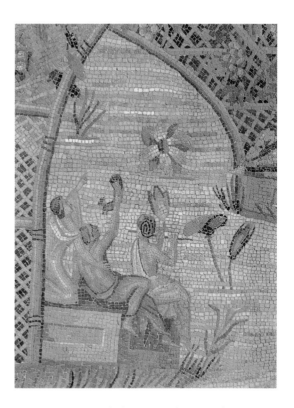

The Romans were famous for their practice and enjoyment of massage and bathing with scented oils.

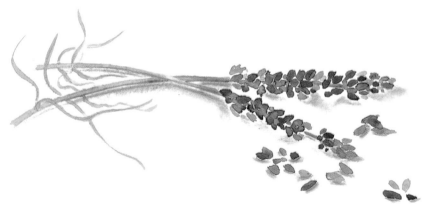

The healing power of lavender was one of the first to be re-discovered.

Native American Indians throughout the northern continent also used aromatic oils and produced their own herbal remedies. These were discovered when the early settlers began to make their way across the plains and prairies of the 'New World'.

However, despite their use in many other world cultures for centuries, it was not until the 19th century that scientists in Europe and Great Britain began researching the effects of essential oils on bacteria in humans. A French chemist, Rene Maurice Gattefosse, began his research into the healing powers of essential oils after burning his hand in his laboratory. Almost without thinking he immersed the burn in lavender oil and was immediately impressed by how quickly the burn healed. In 1937 he published a book about the anti-microbial effects of the oils and it was he who actually coined the word 'Aromatherapy'. He went on to set up a business producing oils for use in fragrances and cosmetics. At around the same time another Frenchman, Albert Couvreur, published a book on the medicinal uses of essential oils.

A French medical doctor, Jean Valnet, discovered Gattefosse's research and began experimenting with essential oils. At about the same time Margaret Maury, a French biochemist, developed a unique method of applying these oils to the skin with massage. Micheline Arcier, now living in London, studied and worked with Maury and Valnet and their combined techniques created the form of Aromatherapy that is now used all over the world.

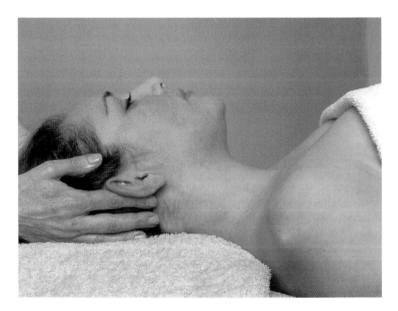

Today aromatherapy is valued throughout the world.

the holistic Approach to health

The holistic approach to keeping healthy is not new. The ancient healing traditions of India and China are based on the idea that the body, mind and spirit form an integrated whole and are inextricably connected with the environment. These traditions further maintain that to be healthy, all of these elements must exist in a dynamically balanced state of well-being.

"The cure of the part should not be attempted without treatment of the whole. No attempt should be made to cure the body without the soul. If the body and head are to be healthy you must begin by curing the mind. Let no one persuade you to cure the head until he has first given you his soul to be cured."

Plato 427-347 BC

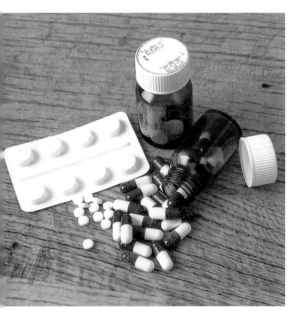

Aromatherapy complements conventional medicines, which generally only treat a specific area or set of symptoms.

The human organism can, in theory, be divided into three levels: physical, emotional and mental. However, in reality these are not separate and there is constant interaction between them. If there is imbalance in one level, then the others can not be in harmony. This is in direct contrast with conventional medicine, which treats a particular part of the body, or a particular set of symptoms to cure an ailment, and which normally uses chemical intervention or surgery.

A physical symptom such as a headache may be related to an underlying psychological problem and although dealing with the physical symptom alone may relieve the pain temporarily, it will not necessarily bring about a long-term solution.

Today, more and more people are returning to a holistic lifestyle, as they find that the traditional methods and practises help them to enjoy a higher level of vitality and well-being. Aromatherapy is one holistic practice that can easily be incorporated into our everyday lives to help us achieve a state of well-being.

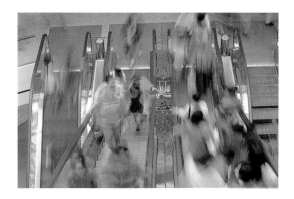

Although some stress is essential in our lives, the stress created in today's environment is often extreme, and detrimental to our well-being.

STRESS

The word stress is one which is familiar to most of us. It is an almost expected part of daily life, and it is hardly surprising to learn that an estimated 75% of visits to GPs are due to stress-related problems.

However, we cannot avoid stress as it is essential to life. It is the dynamic, creative force which makes us sit, walk, run etc. and is therefore vital for our very existence. Stress is the adaptive response of the body to demands made on it. We are all unique and what may be creative stress for one person may be destructive to another. Creative stress can be defined as stress that we can use to inspire us, or to drive us to greater heights or successes, whether personal or professional. Destructive stress on the other hand makes us ill, ruins our concentration and makes us feel as if life is too much for us to deal with.

Although it is true, therefore, that we all need a certain amount of stress in our lives, it is our response to stress that dictates whether a positive or negative effect on our well-being.

In times of fast-moving, constantly changing lifestyles, we are being expected to cope with any demands placed on us and illness or disease is often the only way for our body to tell us that it cannot cope with such pressure. When stress becomes a regular feature in our lives, our energy reserves become rapidly depleted, and if we do not take the time to 'recharge our batteries', then nature often steps in, manifesting some form of illness that forces us to stop and review our lives.

High blood pressure, strokes and heart disease are often considered to be related to stress and other disorders such as rheumatism, cancer, skin disorders and digestive problems are more likely to develop when our resistance is low.

Any change in our lives is potentially stressful as change requires us to adapt. Major changes such as marriage, divorce, new job, redundancy, financial problems or a birth or death in the family are just some of the most common life changes that force us to make major adjustments. If more than one of these changes occur within a short space of time we may overlook the need to take time to adjust. Our response to increased pressure, whether external or self-imposed usually makes us force ourselves to keep going, even when our bodies may be telling us we need to rest or relax. It is this denial of our physical and emotional needs that often results in unpleasant consequences, such as illness, depression or exhaustion.

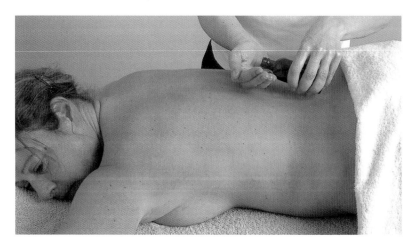

Massage is one of the most effective relaxation techniques. Combined with soothing aromatherapy oils its benefits are increased.

It is therefore very important that we equip ourselves with ways of managing stress. One of the most effective and agreeable methods of doing this is the practise of Aromatherapy, where the use of essential oils plays a vital role.

Conventional medicine often has little to offer when it comes to dealing with stress-related conditions as it usually only treats the symptoms of such problems – emotional distress or insomnia are common examples – with the use of tranquillisers or sleeping tablets. These may help in the short-term, but they are not a long-term solution to the problem.

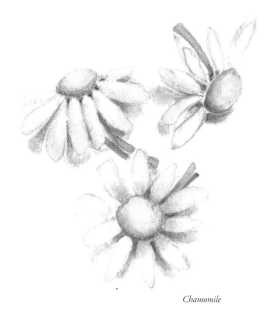

Chamomile

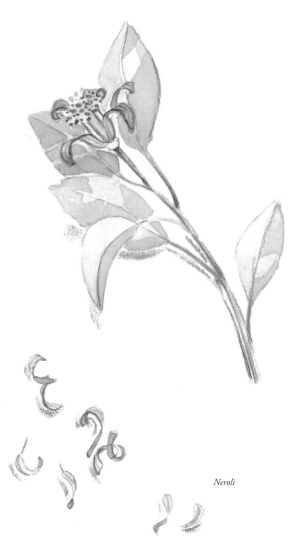

Neroli

As a holistic form of treatment, aromatherapy aims to deal with the underlying cause of the complaint, as well as the symptoms, and this form of treatment is very important when dealing with stress-related problems, as a physical symptom is more often than not a manifestation of an underlying psychological or emotional problem. Essential oils have many properties which make them ideal for helping you to cope with stress. Oils such as chamomile help to relax the body and improve sleep. Neroli is ideal for helping with anxiety and depression, while lavender is helpful for high blood pressure, insomnia and depression. These oils can be used in different ways to help with stress related problems, although one of the easiest, yet most enjoyable methods is to simply relax in a warm bath with essential oils.

Certain oils such as lavender, sandalwood and tea-tree have a positive effect on the immune system, making our bodies more able to cope with the demands and pressures of everyday life. Using these oils on a regular basis can help to prevent stress-related ailments. It is clear, then, that with the help of these wonderful oils, managing the stress in our lives can become easier.

an introduction to
Essential Oils

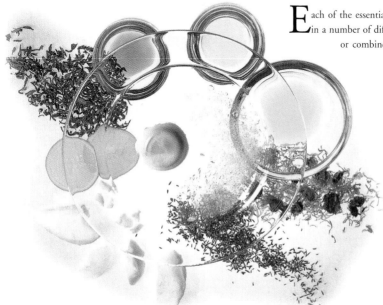

Aromatherapy essential oils can be used in a number of different ways, from healing to cosmetic.

Each of the essential oils used in Aromatherapy can be used in a number of different ways, and can be used either alone or combined with other oils to enhance our health and sense of well-being. Before beginning to use Aromatherapy treatments, it is important to understand how each oil works, and which can be used most effectively to ease or prevent specific ills, or to promote a particular feeling.

Essential oils are highly fragrant, non-oily plant essences. The term oil is somewhat inappropriate as these essences have a consistency which resembles water more than oil. They are volatile and evaporate easily so they must be stored in a cool place, in dark coloured bottles away from direct sunlight.

The essences are insoluble in water but dissolve in vegetable oils, wax and alcohol. The essential oils can be found in different parts of the plant such as the flowers, twigs, leaves and bark, but also often in the rind of the fruit. Each oil originates in special sacs in the plant material.

Essential oils are antiseptic as well as having their own individual properties and have many complex chemical constituents. Due to its many different components one oil can have a variety of uses.

The oils work in various ways on the body. If applied to the skin they are absorbed quickly through the hair follicles due to their molecular structure. They diffuse into the blood stream or are taken up by the lymphatic fluids and transported throughout the body. Different oils are absorbed at different rates and this can vary between 20 minutes to two hours or even more so it is best not to shower for a time after applying the oils.

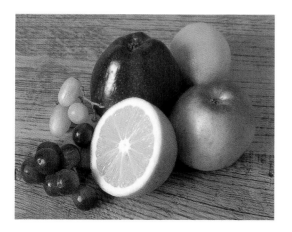

The essential oils are extracted from various parts of the plant. In fruit, oils generally come from rinds or seeds

Before using an oil, it is always very important to note the contra-indications for each oil and to stick closely to these recommendations.

A general rule when choosing oils is to select and use those whose scents you find particularly appealing. The whole principle of Aromatherapy is that it should be a pleasurable experience, and choosing an oil whose aroma is unpleasant to you will not be beneficial. There will generally be more than one oil you can use for a particular purpose, so you shoud be able to find one you like.

The nose plays an important part in Aromatherapy. When inhaling essential oils the odour molecules are transmitted to the emotional centre of the brain known as the limbic system. This system is connected to other parts of the brain involved with memory, breathing and blood circulation as well as the endocrine glands which regulate hormone levels in the body.

The effect on the memory is important as it can help bring back recollections of the past, not all of which will be pleasant. If you do not like the smell of a particular oil, for example, it could well be that it reminds you of something in your past that you would prefer to forget. This is another reason it is a good idea to avoid the use of this oil.

Essential oils are often described as having top, middle or base notes and this relates to the amount of time that the aroma of each oil will last.

- Oils with base notes have the longest lasting aroma, with scents that can last up to one week.

- Oils with middle notes have a shorter span, with aromas lasting about two to three days.

- Oils with top notes have the shortest-lasting aromas, with scents which only last for up to 24 hours.

In terms of creating a balanced perfume, a combination of top, middle and base notes will produce the best results. However, when it comes to making aromatherapy blends, it is not necessary to stick to any fixed rules. As you become familiar with the different oils you will be able to create blends which are right for you. Experimenting with these wonderful essences will be an enjoyable and educational experience, as you learn which oils combine the best, and produce the best effects.

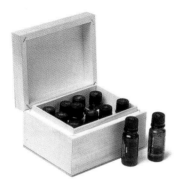

There are many scents to choose from, so finding an aroma that suits you should be easy.

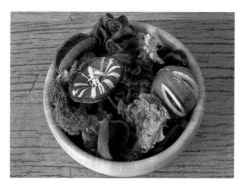

Once you have found the scents you prefer, you can use them in your everyday life in pot pourris for example.

SAFETY PRECAUTIONS

Although essential oils are generally considered to be safe to use they are very powerful, highly concentrated substances which should be treated with a certain amount of respect. It is important to take note of the following safety guidelines before proceeding:

- Do not use any oil that you are not familiar with.

- The following oils should not be used during pregnancy or when breast feeding:
  Thyme, Sage, Wintergreen, Basil, Clove, Marjoram, Cinnamon, Fennel, Jasmine, Juniper, Rosemary, Aniseed, Peppermint, Clary Sage, Oregano, Nutmeg, Bay, Hops, Valerian, Tarragon, Cedarwood.

- The following should be avoided during the first 3 months of pregnancy:
  Chamomile, Geranium, Lavender and Rose.

- If there is history of previous miscarriage do not massage.

- The following oils may cause slight skin irritation:
  Basil, Rosemary, Fennel, Verbena and Lemon Grass.

The only essential oils which can be used undiluted on the skin are Lavender and Tea Tree but care should be taken as some people have a sensitivity to these oils.

- The following oils should NOT be applied to the skin before sunbathing or using a sun-bed:
  Bergamot, Orange, Lemon or other citrus oils.

- If you or anyone you are considering treating, suffer from epilepsy, great care should be taken as certain oils could aggravate the condition. The following oils should NOT be used:
  Fennel, Hyssop, Sage, and Rosemary.

- Do NOT take essential oils internally, although herbal teas can be used in moderation.

- Keep oils away from children and if any essential oil gets in the eye, rinse immediately with water.

- If you are taking homeopathic remedies, check that the essential oil will not interfere with their effectiveness.

- If you have sensitive skin or are prone to allergies you should do a skin patch test before using a particular oil. First wash and dry the forearm, then add a few drops of the blended oil to the gauze of a large plaster. The plaster should be placed on the forearm and left for 24 hours. The plaster should then be removed and if the area appears irritated or red do not use that particular blend. This test does not guarantee that there will not be an adverse reaction but it will give a good indication.

- If you dislike the smell of a particular oil, this is a good indication that the oil is not right for you and a suitable alternative should be used.

- Do not use steam inhalations if you suffer from asthma.

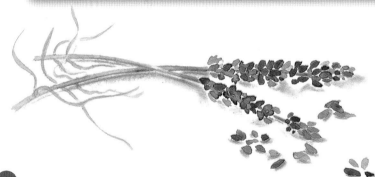

The following pages cover 35 of the most commonly-used Essential oils. Each plant is listed alphabetically by its botanical name, which is shown in brackets after the common name.

CHAMOMILE, ROMAN *(ANTHEMIS NOBILIS)*

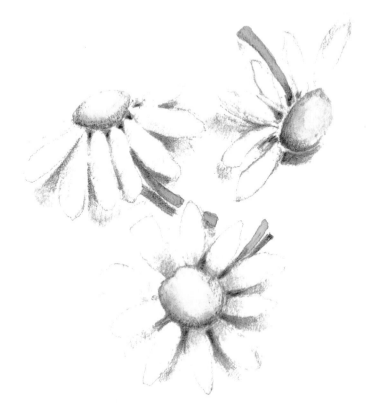

Effects: Soothing and harmonising
Aroma: Middle note

This small plant, native to Europe, has a daisy-like flower. It is mainly cultivated in Italy, England, France and the USA. Chamomile tea is renowned worldwide for its calming effect.

Properties
- Tonic
- Soothing
- Pain reliever
- Antibacterial
- Antiseptic
- Digestive stimulant

Contra-indications
Not to be used during early pregnancy. May cause skin irritation.

Extraction
Steam distillation of the flower heads.

Uses
- Rheumatism
- Gout
- Skin conditions
- Inflammations such as eczema
- Nervous tension
- Neuralgia
- Digestive problems such as colitis and gastritis
- Headaches
- Depression

Chamomile also promotes relaxation and eases tension, anxiety and fear. It has a soothing effect on skin conditions such as ulcers, boils and blisters and may help in conditions such as psoriasis, dermatitis and acne.

Massaging the abdomen is helpful when treating indigestion and flatulence. May help with Irritable Bowel Syndrome.

Chamomile is also very helpful when used in massage to alleviate nervous tension and headaches and lower back pain.

Scent
Sweet, herbal , fruity scent.

Combines with:
- Bergamot
- Geranium
- Lavender
- Clary Sage

FRANKINCENSE *(BOSWELLIA CARTERI)*

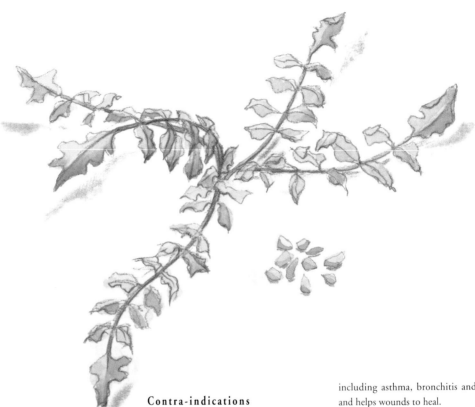

Effects: Uplifting
Aroma: Base/middle note

This small tree is native to the Red Sea area and the oil is produced in China, Somalia and Ethiopia. The spice is used during religious ceremonies and an ingredient in cosmetics.

Properties
- Analgesic
- Anti-inflammatory
- Antiseptic
- Antidepressant
- Expectorant

Contra-indications
None.

Extraction
Steam distillation of the gum resin obtained from the bark of the trees.

Uses
- Skin care
- Respiratory conditions
- Urinary infections
- Nervous conditions

Frankincense also has a beneficial effect on mature skins.

It can be used blended as a chest and back massage for respiratory conditions including asthma, bronchitis and colds, and helps wounds to heal.

It is a uterine tonic and can be helpful for heavy periods and also as a massage after birth.

It is helpful as a blended massage oil for those who are frightened and nervous and is very comforting for those who feel isolated and alone.

Scent
Sweet, warm and balsamic.

Combines with:
- Rose
- Sandalwood
- Lavender
- Neroli

YLANG YLANG (CANANGIUM ODORATUM)

Effects: Stimulating
Aroma: Base/middle note

This tall tree is native to the Philippines and the Far East. The large distinctive flowers can be various colours but the yellow ones are considered to produce the best oil.

Properties
- Antiseptic
- Antidepressant
- Calming
- Sedative

Contra-indications
May be an irritant to sensitive skins and should not be used on inflammatory skin conditions. The strong scent can cause headaches.

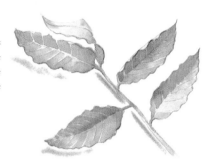

Extraction
Steam distillation of the flowers.

Uses
- Intestinal infections
- High blood pressure
- Stress

Ylang-Ylang is helpful in dealing with anxiety, panic and shock as it has a relaxing effect on the nervous system. It is also believed to help feelings of resentment, guilt and jealousy.

It has a balancing effect on the hormones and is a tonic for the uterus.

Ylang-Ylang oil has a balancing effect on oily and dry skins.

Scent
Powerful, sweet, balsamic, floral, exotic.

Combines with:
- Clary Sage
- Geranium
- Lavender
- Lemon
- Cedarwood

CEDARWOOD (CEDRUS ATLANTICA)

Effects: Strengthening and powerful
Aroma: Base note

This tree grows in southern Europe, the Orient and North America. Cedarwood gum was used by the Egyptians many years ago as an important ingredient in the mummifying process.

Properties
- Antiseptic
- Sedative
- Expectorant
- Antifungal
- Astringent

Contra-indications
May irritate sensitive skins. Do not use during pregnancy.

Extraction
Steam distillation of the wood as well as the sawdust.

Uses:
- Bronchitis

- Nervous tension
- Cellulite
- Cystitis
- Certain skin conditions such as eczema.

Cedarwood is good for acne, and oily skin and when blended with rosemary and eucalyptus is used as a treatment for dandruff. It has a calming effect on the nervous system. May be helpful for arthritic and rheumatic pains.

Scent
Woody.

Combines with:
- Bergamot
- Rosemary
- Sandalwood

NEROLI/ORANGE BLOSSOM *(CITRUS AURANTIUM)*

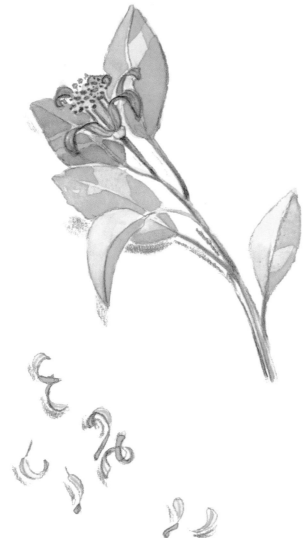

Extraction
Steam distillation of the flowers.

Uses
* Flatulence
* Headaches
* Nervous tension
* Depression
* Insomnia.

Neroli is also used in skin preparations.

Due to its very soothing effect, Neroli is very helpful in stress-related conditions such as panic attacks and irritable bowel syndrome when used diluted in massage.

It has a calming effect on the heart and has a beneficial effect on dry, sensitive skin and broken capillaries. Being antispasmodic it is helpful in digestive problems such as colitis.

Scent
Rich, floral, refreshing.

Combines with:
* Lavender
* Chamomile
* Sandalwood
* Citrus oils

Effects: Calming and peaceful
Aroma: Top note

An evergreen tree with fragrant white blossom which originated in the Far East. It is now grown in the Midi region of France, Southern Italy, Spain, Mexico, California and South America.

Properties
* Antidepressant
* Antiseptic
* Antispasmodic
* Sedative

Contra-indications
None.

ORANGE (CITRUS AURANTIUM)

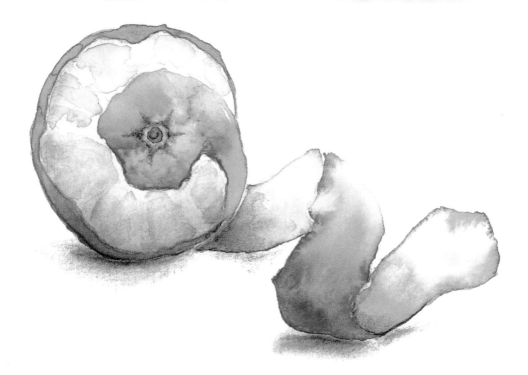

Effects: Calming and energising

Aroma: Top note

This is the same tree that produces Neroli oil — an evergreen tree with fragrant white blossom which originated in the Far East. The orange tree is a familiar sight in the Mediterranean regions with blossom appearing in Spring and Autumn.

Properties
- Antidepressant
- Antiseptic
- Antispasmodic
- Digestive
- Detoxifying
- Sedative
- Tonic

Contra-indications
May irritate skin and is photo toxic.

Extraction
Expression of the rind of the fruit.

Uses
- Anxiety
- Mature skins
- Indigestion
- Muscular pains
- Cellulite

Orange has a beneficial effect on the nervous system, as it calms and relaxes and may help insomnia.

Orange is beneficial for digestive problems such as constipation, diarrhoea and flatulence, and helps the system eliminate toxins through the skin. Orange can also relieve muscular aches and pains.

It is beneficial for dry skin and dermatitis but should only be used in very low dilutions.

Respiratory conditions can be alleviated, and orange is a useful oil for depression and sadness.

Scent
Fresh and light. Fruity and sweet.

Combines with:
- Frankincense
- Sandalwood
- Lavender
- Rosemary
- Ylang-ylang

BERGAMOT *(CITRUS BERGAMIA)*

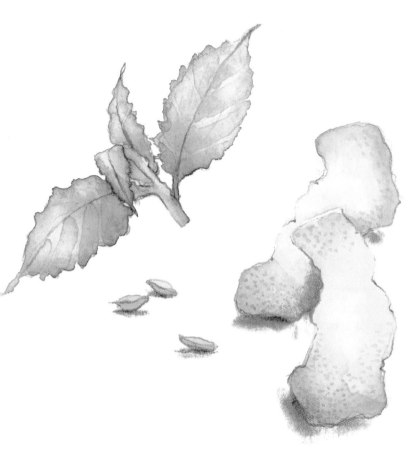

Extraction
Expression of the outer part of the peel from the small orange-like fruit.

Uses
- Sore throat
- Loss of appetite
- Flatulence
- Its antiseptic properties are helpful in the treatment of acne and also for boils and abscesses.
- It can also help to ease shingles, chicken pox and cold sores.
- It has a positive effect on the immune system and is helpful for colds, flu, mouth infections and sore throats.
- It is a useful air freshener when used in a vaporiser.
- It can be added to a bath in a well-diluted form to alleviate both cystitis and thrush.

Bergamot is also widely used in perfumes and the confection industry. It is used to flavour Earl Grey Tea and has a positive effect on anxiety and depression.

Scent
Fruity with slightly balsamic, spicy undertone. Fresh and sharp.

Effects: Uplifting and refreshing
Aroma: Top note

This small tree is native to Morocco and parts of Asia. The name comes from a small town in Italy called Bergamo where the oil was first sold. Bergamot belongs to the same family as the orange tree and one of its more familiar uses is as the flavouring in Earl Grey tea.

Properties
- Antiseptic
- Antispasmodic
- Antidepressant
- Uplifting

Contra-indications
Bergamot is photo toxic so should not be used with exposure to sunlight.

Combines with:
- Chamomile
- Juniper
- Neroli

PETITGRAIN (CITRUS BIGARDIA)

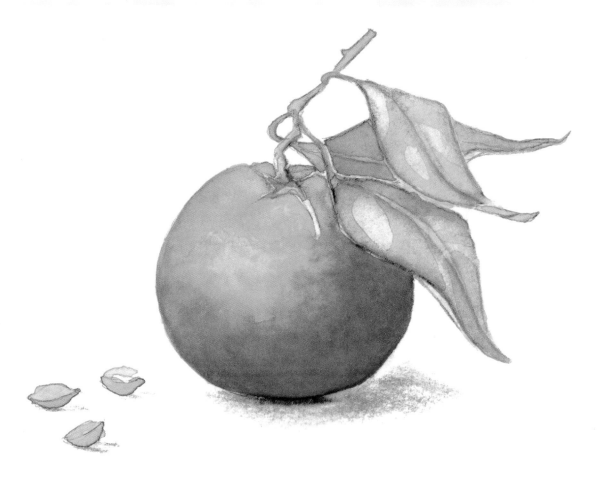

Effects: Restoring

Aroma: Top note

This is yet another oil produced from the Orange tree.

Properties

- Antibacterial
- Antifungal
- Antiseptic
- Antispasmodic
- Stimulant

Contra-indications

None.

Extraction

Steam distillation of the twigs and leaves.

Uses

- Respiratory infections
- Skin conditions such as acne.

Petitgrain is also beneficial in digestive conditions such as flatulence.

It has a positive effect on the nervous system and is helpful in cases of stress, depression, nervous exhaustion and stress-induced insomnia.

Scent

Fresh, sweet, floral.

Combines with:

- Other citrus oils

23

LEMON (CITRUS LIMONOM)

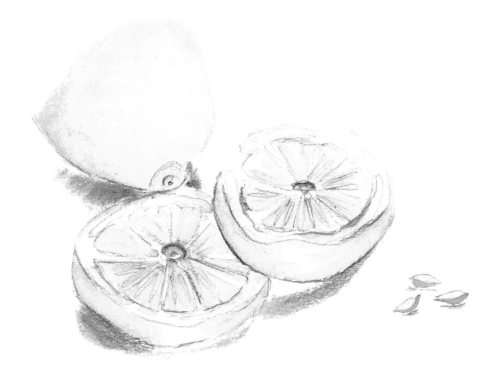

Effects: Cleansing and stimulating

Aroma: Top note

This evergreen tree is thought to have originated in India, and now grows extensively in southern Europe, particularly in Portugal and Spain.

Properties
- Antiseptic
- Astringent
- Antiviral
- Stimulant

Contra-indications
May irritate sensitive skin. Photo toxic.

Extraction
Expression of the outer part of the rind of the fruit.

Uses
- Sinusitis
- Sore throat
- Tonsillitis
- Inflammation of the gums
- Migraine
- Chilblains
- Verrucae

Lemon is also a good first aid treatment for snake and insect bites. Also has a great use in skin and beauty care as a skin tonic and helps clear warts, corns and verrucae.

It has a general cleansing effect on the body. Lemon may be effective in relieving headaches and rheumatic pains.

It can be used in a vaporiser but should NOT be inhaled and sun and sun beds should be avoided for several hours after use on the skin.

Scent
Refreshing, clean, lively.

Combines with:
- Chamomile
- Frankincense
- Lavender
- Sandalwood
- Ylang-Ylang
- Other citrus oils

GRAPEFRUIT *(CITRUS PARADISI)*

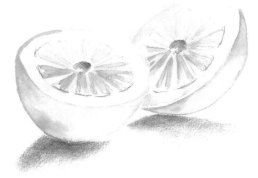

Effects: Refreshing
Aroma: Top note

A tree native to the West Indies and Asia and cultivated in California, Brazil and Israel.

Properties
- Antiseptic
- Astringent
- Diuretic
- Stimulant

Contra-indications
Grapefruit is photo toxic.

Extraction
Expression of the peel of the fruit.

Uses
- Digestive problems
- Water retention
- Depression
- Anxiety, self doubt

Combined with lemon, grapefruit can make a refreshing and revitalising morning bath.

Scent
Sweet, fresh, citrus-y.

Combines with:
- Lavender
- Other citrus oils

MYRRH *(COMMIPHORA MYRRHA)*

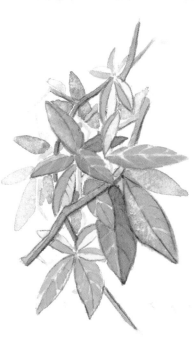

Effects: Toning
Aroma: Middle note

This bush is native to Africa and Arabia. The oil has been used since ancient times.

Properties
- Analgesic
- Astringent
- Antiseptic
- Expectorant

Contra-indications
None.

Extraction
Steam distillation of the gum resin.

Uses
- Arthritis
- Coughs and colds
- Bronchitis
- Stimulates digestive system

Scent
Warm and spicy.

Combines with:
- Frankincense
- Orange
- Geranium
- Pine

CYPRESS (CUPRESSUS SEMPERVIRENS)

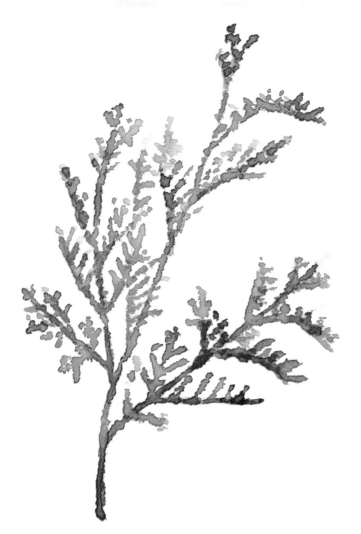

Extraction
Steam distillation of both the needles and twigs.

Uses:
- Rheumatism
- Muscle and nervous tension
- Haemorrhoids
- Spasmodic coughs

Cypress is helpful as a massage oil to treat rheumatic aches and pains as well as swollen joints.

Used as an inhalant, its antispasmodic properties help alleviate coughs, bronchitis, asthma and sore throats.

Cypress is very helpful for regulating the menstrual cycle and treating oedema. It also has a beneficial effect on menopause symptoms such as hot flushes and irritability.

It can be used in treating oily skin and hair.

Scent
Refreshing and sweet.

Combines with:
- Citrus oils
- Lavender
- Sandalwood
- Rose
- Juniper

Effects: Refreshing

Aroma: Middle/base note

This is a tall evergreen tree native to the Mediterranean regions. It is now cultivated in France, Spain and Morocco. It was used as a natural remedy by many of the ancient civilisations.

Properties
- Astringent
- Antispasmodic
- Diuretic
- Expectorant

Contra-indications
Due to its effect on the menstrual cycle, cypress should be avoided in pregnancy.

EUCALYPTUS (*EUCALYPTUS GLOBULUS*)

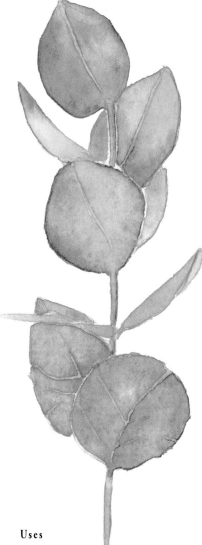

Effects: Balancing and stimulating
Aroma: Top/middle note

This tall evergreen is also known as the Gum Tree and originated in Australia. There are hundreds of varieties, many of which are now found in Southern Europe, Brazil and California.

Properties

- Stimulant
- Antiseptic
- Analgesic
- Antiviral
- Anti-inflammatory
- Decongestant, particularly useful for respiratory as well as urinary tract infections.
- Insect repellent

Contra-indications

Eucalyptus is a powerful oil and should be avoided by sufferers of high blood pressure or epilepsy. It can prove fatal if taken internally.

Extraction

Steam distillation of the leaves and twigs.

Uses

- Sinusitis
- Flu
- Bronchitis
- Sore throat
- Asthma
- Other pulmonary conditions.
- Rheumatism and aching muscles
- Skin problems such as burns, cuts, wounds and ulcers

Eucalyptus is also very useful as an air disinfectant. Burning the oil helps to purify the air in sickrooms.

Used as an inhalant it is beneficial for respiratory conditions and as a chest massage oil using the diluted oil.

Its anti-inflammatory properties are helpful when used as a massage oil to relieve pains and aches associated with rheumatism and arthritis. It is helpful for neuralgia and headaches.

It can be used to alleviate urinary infections such as cystitis when added to a bath.

Scent

Camphorous, woody, clear.

Combines with:

- Lavender
- Rosemary
- Marjoram
- Juniper

CLOVE *(EUGENIA CARYOPHYLLATA)*

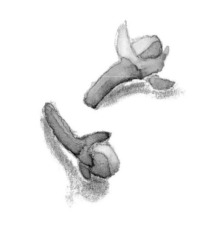

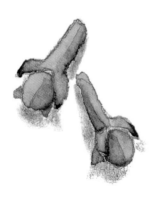

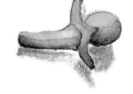

Effects: Warming
Aroma: Base/middle note

This is a small evergreen tree which grows in the West Indies and Madagascar. Cloves are commonly used in cooking and dental preparations.

Properties
- Analgesic
- Expectorant
- Stimulant

Contra-indications
Clove is a very potent oil and should be used with great care. Used for massage it could cause skin irritation. Only use in very low dilutions less than 1%.

Extraction
Steam distillation from both the stalks and stems.

Properties
- Antiseptic
- Analgesic
- Antispasmodic
- Disinfectant
- Insecticide

Uses
- Toothache
- Muscular and nerve tension
- Infected wounds
- Indigestion

Clove also relieves respiratory conditions and has been used to treat bronchitis, laryngitis and colds.

It is an excellent room disinfectant and insect repellent.

Clove is also used in natural toothpastes.

Scent
Sweet, spicy and fresh.

Combines with:
- Lavender
- Orange
- Bergamot
- Ylang-ylang

FENNEL *(FOENICULUM VULGARE)*

Effects: Clearing
Aroma: Middle note

This herb has yellow flowers and originates from Spain and Eastern Europe. It belongs to the carrot family.

Properties
- Antiseptic
- Anti-spasmodic
- Diuretic
- Stimulant

Contra-indications
May irritate sensitive skins. Do not use in pregnancy or with epilepsy sufferers.

Extraction
Steam distillation of the seeds.

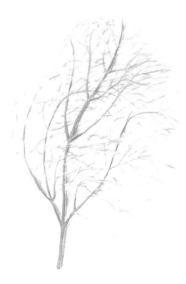

Uses
- Indigestion
- Flatulence
- Nervous tension

Its diuretic properties make fennel helpful in the treatment of gout, particularly when combined with juniper.

Useful in digestive problems such as constipation and flatulence. (Fennel tea helps colic and diarrhoea).

Scent
Sweet but earthy.

Combines with:
- Geranium
- Lavender
- Sandalwood

JASMINE *(JASMINUM GRANDIFLORUM)*

Effects: Soothing
Aroma: Base note

This is a shrub native to Asia and India and which is cultivated in China and the Mediterranean regions. It is an evergreen with small, fragrant flowers.

Properties
- Antidepressant
- Antiseptic
- Antispasmodic
- Expectorant

Contra-indications
Generally none but allergic reactions have been known.

Extraction
Solvent extraction of the flowers.

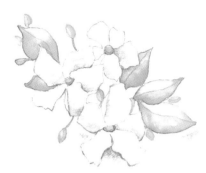

Uses
- Headache
- Anxiety
- Lack of confidence

Jasmine is also helpful for respiratory conditions such as laryngitis, catarrh and coughs.

It can help with uterine disorders such as period pains and labour pains.

It has a beneficial effect on the nervous system and may help ease tension and anxiety.

It is used in skin care and has a beneficial effect on dry or sensitive skins.

Scent
Warm and floral.

Combines with:
- Sandalwood
- Rose
- Chamomile
- Ylang-ylang
- Citrus oils

JUNIPER *(JUNIPERUS COMMUNIS)*

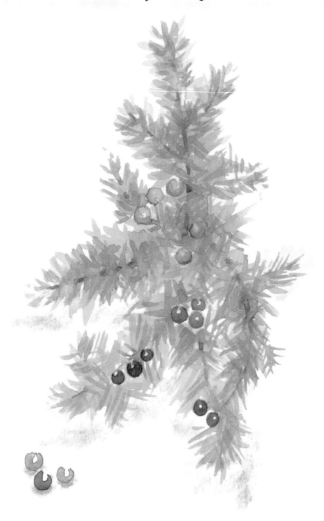

Effects: Cleansing
Aroma: Middle note

This small hardwood bush thrives in Arctic regions and can be found in Sweden, Canada and central Northern Europe. It has been used for many years as an antiseptic.

Properties
- Analgesic
- Astringent
- Diuretic
- Expectorant

Contra-indications
Juniper should not be used by people with severe kidney disease, as it can over-stimulate the kidneys. Avoid use during pregnancy.

Extraction
Steam distillation of the berries.

Uses
- Eczema
- Acne
- Sores and ulcers
- Rheumatism and gout
- Cystitis.

Juniper is also a useful disinfectant.

Use diluted as a massage oil for aches and pains and rheumatism.

Juniper has a calming effect and is helpful to ease stress when used as a massage oil.

It is very helpful in treating gout as it helps with elimination of toxins. Due to its diuretic effect, Juniper is helpful in conditions of the genito-urinary tract such as cystitis.

It may be helpful for acne, dermatitis and weeping eczema and can sometimes help cellulite.

Juniper is very cleansing emotionally as well as physically and helps revitalise.

Scent
Fresh, woody and sweet.

Combines with:
- Lavender
- Rose
- Rosemary
- Frankincense
- Sandalwood

LAVENDER (*LAVENDULA ANGUSTIFOLIA*)

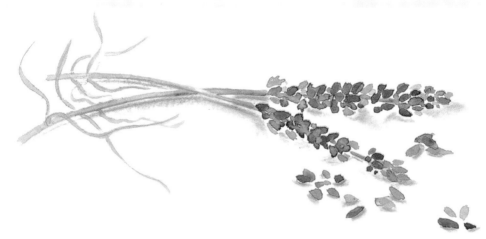

Effects: Calming and healing
Aroma: Middle note

This flowering shrub is native to the Mediterranean regions and is now cultivated worldwide. Its lovely violet-blue flowers are a familiar sight in many English gardens. The highest quality lavender is found growing at high altitudes. Lavender was very popular with the Romans who used it in connection with bathing. Lavender is one of the mildest yet most effective of all the essential oils and probably the most widely used. It is a must for any first aid kit.

Properties
- Analgesic
- Anti-inflammatory
- Antiseptic
- Diuretic
- Sedative
- Calming
- Insecticide

Contra-indications
Avoid use during the early stages of pregnancy. Lavender should be used with caution in cases of low blood pressure.

Extraction
Steam distillation of the flowering tops.

Uses
- Rheumatism
- Skin conditions
- Headaches
- Colds and flu
- Sinusitis
- Bronchitis
- Insomnia
- Burns
- Dandruff
- Wounds and sores, such as leg ulcers and acne.

Lavender is also very useful for treating insect and snake bites. Undiluted lavender oil can be added to burns and is a very effective treatment.

Due to its sedative properties, lavender is very helpful for relieving insomnia and can be used for this purpose diluted in a massage oil, added to a bath or a few drops put on a pillow.

It can be used in a massage blend to ease aches and pains and also added to a bath for this purpose.

It is very helpful in easing headaches by massaging the oil on the temples and the feet.

As an inhalant it relieves respiratory problems such as bronchitis, catarrh, and throat infections.

It is helpful for circulatory conditions such as chilblains.

It has a beneficial effect on tension and anxiety.

As already stated, lavender is very helpful in dealing with minor burns and sunburn, and may also be useful in treating psoriasis and eczema.

Massaging the lower back and abdomen with lavender oil eases period pains. Hot compresses also help.

Scent
Floral, woody, sweet, herbaceous.

Combines with:
- Clary Sage
- Marjoram
- Geranium
- Juniper
- Frankincense

TEA-TREE *(MELALEUCA ALTERNIFOLIA)*

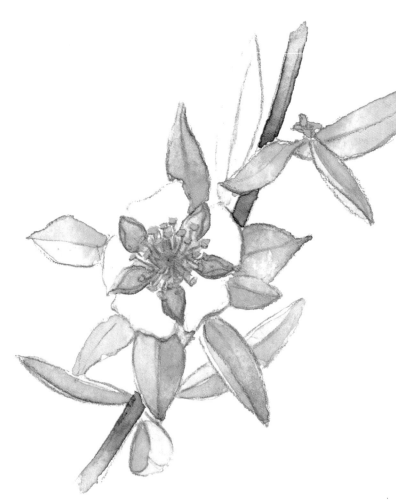

Effects: Cleansing

Aroma: Top note

This tree is a species of the Melaleuca tree found in Queensland and New South Wales in Australia.

Properties
- Powerful antiseptic
- Antifungal
- Antiviral
- Antibiotic
- Detoxifying
- Stimulant
- Insecticide

Contra-indications
May irritate sensitive skins.

Extraction
Steam distillation of the leaves and twigs.

Uses
- Helps the immune system attack infections, viruses, fungi and yeast
- Helpful in colds, flu and catarrh

It is useful for the treatment of athletes foot, corns etc. A few drops can also be added to a foot bath.

Adding the diluted oil of tea tree to a bath will help alleviate urinary problems such as cystitis, and fungal infections such as Candida albicans which is related to thrush.

It has a beneficial effect on skin problems such as spots, burns, warts, sunburn, boils.

Scent
Spicy, fresh, medicinal.

Combines with:
This oil is best not mixed with other essential oils.

CAJEPUT *(MELALEUCA LEUCODENDRON)*

Effects: Clearing
Aroma: Top note

This is a tall tree which grows abundantly in Malaysia and the Philippines. The name means 'white tree'. It comes from the same family as tea-tree.

Properties
- Pain reliever
- Antiseptic
- Expectorant
- Insecticide

Contra-indications
Cajeput may be a skin irritant in high concentrations.

Extraction
Steam distillation of the fresh leaves.

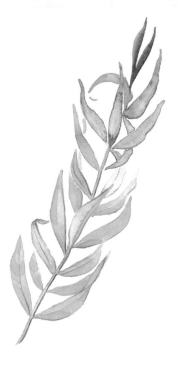

Uses
- Neuralgia
- Rheumatism
- Lung congestion
- Toothache
- Earache
- Colds
- Skin conditions such as acne.

Cajeput is also good for massaging tired muscles and joints.
    It can be used as an inhalation for laryngitis and bronchitis.

Scent
Medicinal camphorous smell.

Combines with:
- Eucalyptus
- Rosemary
- Tea-tree

MELISSA/LEMON BALM *(MELISSA OFFICINALIS)*

Effects: Calming
Aroma: Middle note

A bushy herb with pink or white flowers, native to the Mediterranean regions.

Properties
- Antidepressant
- Antispasmodic
- Sedative

Contra-indications
May cause skin irritation so always use well-diluted. It is difficult to find pure .

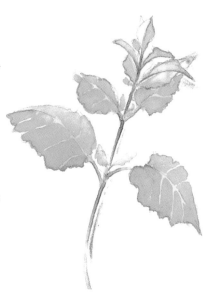

Extraction
Steam distillation of the leaves and tops.

Uses
- Colds and flu

Melissa has a beneficial effect on the nervous system and is helpful in stress related conditions.

Scent
Fresh, sweet, herbaceous.

Combines with:
- Bergamot
- Geranium
- Eucalyptus

PEPPERMINT (*MENTHA PIPERITA*)

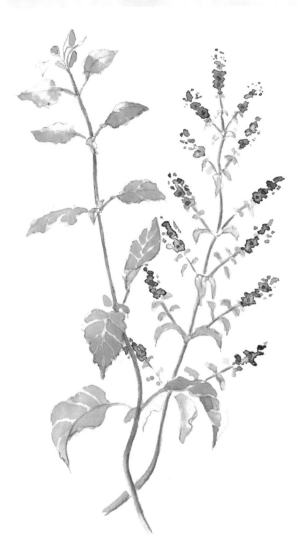

- Astringent
- Decongestant
- Expectorant
- Digestive aid

Contra-indications

Peppermint could irritate sensitive skins, and is not ideal for use in full body massage. However, it can be helpful in localised areas.

Extraction

Steam distillation of leaves and the flowering top.

Uses

- Asthma
- Bronchitis
- Sinusitis
- Migraine
- Indigestion and other digestive problems.

Peppermint is also useful as an insect repellent, and is particularly effective against mosquitoes.

Massage the diluted oil into the temples to ease headaches. Steam inhalations are helpful for respiratory problems.

Massaging the abdomen will help relieve colic and indigestion.

Added to a bowl of water, peppermint is excellent for refreshing tired feet.

Helpful in treating muscular and joint pains.

Effects: Stimulating

Aroma: Top note

This herb has been used for many centuries as a medicine, particularly in the treatment of digestive problems. It is grown widely in France, Italy, America and England. The leaves can be used to make peppermint tea which is believed to aid digestion.

Properties
- Antiseptic
- Antispasmodic
- Analgesic

Scent
Fresh, strong, grassy, minty.

Combines with:
- Eucalyptus
- Rosemary

BASIL *(OCIMUM BASILICUM)*

Effects: Uplifting and stimulating
Aroma: Top note

This herb originated in Asia and is used extensively in the traditional Indian medicine known as Ayurveda. The plant is very aromatic and is a popular ingredient in cookery, particularly Italian dishes.

Properties
- Antidepressant
- Antiseptic
- Uplifting
- Analgesic
- Antispasmodic
- Emmenagogue

Contra-indications
May cause irritation to sensitive skins so always use well-diluted. Not to be used during pregnancy.

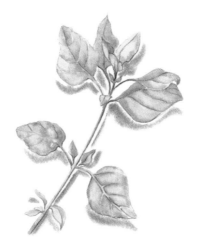

Extraction
Steam distillation of the leaves and flowering tops.

Uses
- Migraine
- Mental fatigue
- Nervous tension
- Sinus congestion
- Bronchitis
- Colds
- Constipation
- Rheumatism.

Can also be used in the first aid treatment of wasp stings and snake bites.

Scent
Fresh, sweet and spicy.

Combines with:
- Frankincense
- Geranium
- Citrus oils

MARJORAM *(ORIGANUM MAJORANA)*

Effects: Soothing and warming
Aroma: Middle note

A bushy plant native to France, Spain, Hungary and Yugoslavia. It has very small white flowers.

Properties
- Analgesic,
- Antiseptic
- Antispasmodic
- Diuretic

Contra-indications
Not to be used during pregnancy.

Extraction
Steam distillation of the leaves and flowering tops.

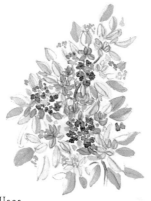

Uses
- Anxiety
- Bronchitis
- Insomnia
- Aches and pains
- Sinusitis
- PMT

Marjoram has a beneficial effect on rheumatism, arthritis, sprains and cramp.

It can also help relieve digestive problems such as colic, flatulence and constipation, and can be used to relieve skin problems and bruises.

Respiratory conditions such as bronchitis can be alleviated.

Scent
Warm, spicy, woody.

Combines with:
- Bergamot
- Cedarwood
- Lavender
- Rosemary

GERANIUM (PELARGONIUM GRAVEOLENS)

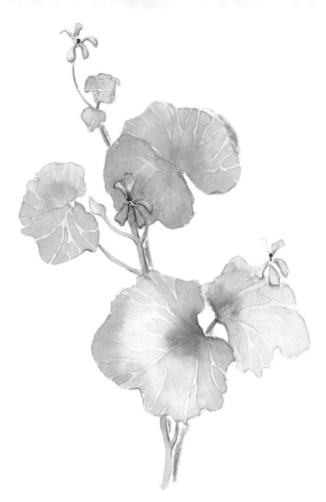

Effects: Comforting and healing

Aroma: Middle note

This shrub originated in Algeria, Madagascar and Guinea. There are hundreds of different species of the Geranium family. It has a colourful flower in varying shades of pink and is a familiar sight in window boxes, particularly in the Mediterranean regions.

Properties
- Antiseptic
- Antifungal
- Anti-spasmodic
- Diuretic

Contra-indications
Geranium oil may irritate sensitive skins. It is best avoided during pregnancy.

Extraction
Steam distillation of the flowers, stalks and leaves.

Uses
- Neuralgia
- Tonsillitis
- Inflammation of the breasts
- Slow circulation
- Burns
- Oedema of the legs
- Rheumatism

Geranium is also helpful in dealing with PMT and menopause symptoms. Its diuretic properties make geranium useful for helping with fluid retention.

Used in massage or inhalations, geranium has a beneficial effect on nervous tension and depression. Massaging with the diluted oil also helps poor circulation. It has a soothing effect on inflamed tissue and can ease swollen legs and oedema. Its astringent quality makes geranium ideal as a skin tonic and conditions such as burns and eczema may respond well to it.

Scent
Floral, earthy and sweet.

Combines with:
- Lavender
- Chamomile
- Rosemary
- Sandalwood
- Cypress
- Juniper

PINE (PINUS SYLVESTRIS)

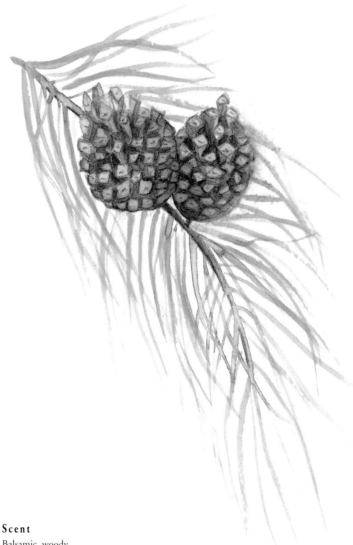

Effects: Clearing
Aroma: Middle note

This tall evergreen is found extensively in Scandinavia, the former Soviet Union and Europe. There are many species of pine but the needles of the Scotch Pine are considered to produce the best oil.

Properties
- Antiseptic
- Expectorant
- Tonic

Contra-indications
May cause irritation to sensitive skins.

Extraction
Steam distillation of the needles.

Uses
- Respiratory tract infections
- Flu
- Sinusitis
- Rheumatism
- Gout

Pine is also useful as a disinfectant.

It is ideal as an inhalation for the treatment of respiratory problems such as bronchitis and laryngitis.

As a massage oil, use diluted to ease aches and pain such as gout and rheumatism. It can also be used as a compress in these conditions.

Burnt in a vaporiser pine is ideal as a room disinfectant.

Scent
Balsamic, woody.

Combines with:
- Eucalyptus
- Sandalwood
- Lavender
- Geranium
- Rosemary

BLACK PEPPER *(PIPER NIGRUM)*

Effects: Stimulating
Aroma: Middle note

This is a woody climbing vine native to India. The oil is also produced in Malaysia and China.

Properties
- Expectorant
- Diuretic
- Stimulant

Contra-indications
Use in low dilutions as this oil may irritate sensitive skins. Avoid during the first three months of pregnancy.

Extraction
Steam distillation of the black peppercorns.

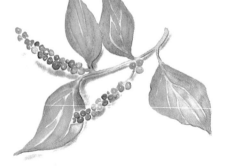

Uses
- Indigestion
- Sinus congestion
- Helpful for chilblains
- Colds and flu
- It is beneficial for digestive problems such as heartburn, flatulence and constipation and can also help in cases of loss of appetite.
- Muscular aches and pains

Scent
Warm and peppery.

Combines with:
- Lavender
- Sandalwood
- Rosemary

PATCHOULI (POGOSTEMON CABLIN)

Effects: Soothing
Aroma: Base note

A flowering herb native to Asia.

Properties
- Antiseptic
- Anti-inflammatory
- Astringent
- Diuretic
- Sedative
- Antidepressant

Contra-indications
None.

Extraction
Steam distillation of the dried leaves.

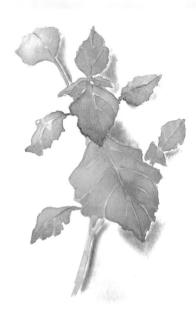

Uses
- Anxiety
- Skin conditions such as eczema, acne, scar tissue and chapped skin

Patchouli can have a beneficial effect on athlete's foot.

Due to its diuretic effect, patchouli may be an effective treatment for water retention and cellulite.

Scent
Sweet, woody.

Combines with:
- Lemon
- Neroli
- Lavender
- Ylang Ylang

ROSE (*ROSA CENTIFOLIA /ROSA DAMASCENA*)

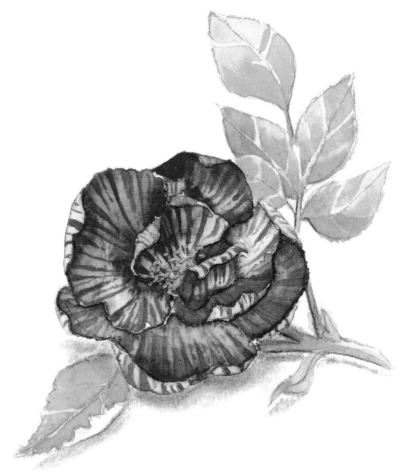

Effects: Comforting
Aroma: Base/middle note

We are all familiar with this beautiful plant. Roses are cultivated in Bulgaria, Turkey and Morocco. It is one of the most useful essential oils but unfortunately it is extremely expensive. Distillation of roses originated many years ago in ancient Persia.

Properties
- Antidepressant
- Antiseptic
- Antispasmodic
- Astringent
- Diuretic
- Sedative
- Antibacterial

Contra-indications
Avoid using rose during the early stages of pregnancy.

Extraction
Distillation of the flower petals.

Uses
- Headache
- Sore throat
- Insomnia
- Depression

Rose water is used extensively in skin care.
Massage with the blended oil will help depression, pre-menstrual tension and regulation of the menstrual cycle.

It has a beneficial effect on mature, dry and sensitive skins as well as broken thread veins.

Scent
Warm, rich, floral, intense.

Combines with:
- Chamomile
- Lavender
- Sandalwood
- Jasmine
- Bergamot
- Geranium

ROSEMARY (*ROSEMARINUS OFFICINALIS*)

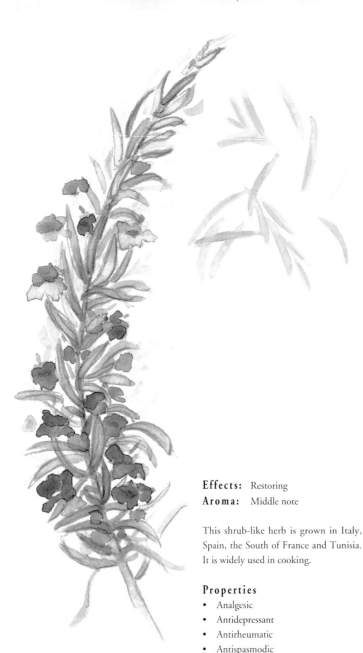

Effects: Restoring
Aroma: Middle note

This shrub-like herb is grown in Italy, Spain, the South of France and Tunisia. It is widely used in cooking.

Properties

- Analgesic
- Antidepressant
- Antirheumatic
- Antispasmodic
- Diuretic
- Stimulant
- Decongestant
- Antiseptic

Contra-indications

As rosemary is highly stimulating, it should not be used in cases of epilepsy, high blood pressure and pregnancy.

Extraction

Steam distillation of the flowering top.

Uses

- Rheumatism
- Gout
- Liver and gall bladder problems
- Colds and flu
- Wounds and burns
- General fatigue
- Digestive problems

Rosemary is also used extensively in cooking. Rosemary is said to help memory and is often used by students during exams by adding a drop to a tissue.

Used as a blend in massage it helps relieve aches and pains and improves circulation. As a rub before and after sports activities Rosemary helps maintain suppleness. Massaging the chest with diluted oil alleviates cold symptoms.

Due to its diuretic effect, Rosemary may help with water retention, cellulite and menstrual cramps. It has an astringent effect on the skin.

Scent

Refreshing, herbaceous, woody.

Combines with:

- Cedarwood
- Geranium
- Juniper

CLARY SAGE (SALVIA SCLAREA)

Effects: Soothing and warming
Aroma: Top/middle note

Clary Sage is a herb with small purplish-blue flowers, and is a native of Southern Europe.

Properties
- Antispasmodic
- Antiseptic
- Calming
- Anti-inflammatory
- Sedative, uplifts the spirit

Contra-indications
Due to its highly sedative effect, Clary Sage should not be used before driving. Do not use during pregnancy.

Extraction
Steam distillation of the flowering tops and leaves.

Uses
- Respiratory problems
- Asthma
- Sore throat
- Depression
- Skin preparations

Clary Sage can be used as a massage blend or diluted in the bath. It is an ideal treatment for both nervous exhaustion and depression.

Massaging the abdomen gently will help relieve period pain and other uterine problems. It regulates hormones and may help PMT symptoms. Clary Sage is also good for relieving digestive problems such as wind by massaging the abdomen.

Its general soothing action is excellent for cramp and muscle spasm and it acts like a tonic to the whole body.

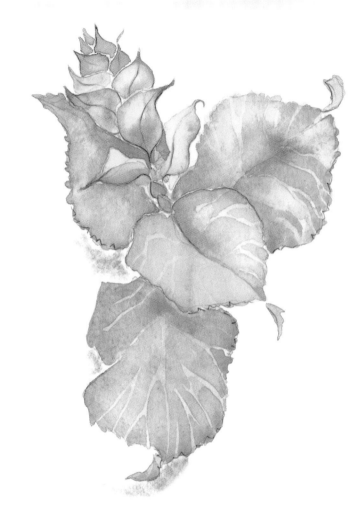

It can also be useful for inflamed, puffy skin and dandruff.

Scent
Sweet, spicy, herbaceous smell.

Combines with:
- Lavender
- Geranium
- Rose
- Rosemary
- Ylang-Ylang

41

SANDALWOOD (SANTALUM ALBUM)

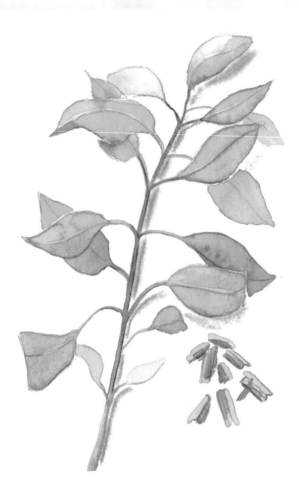

Effects: Balancing

Aroma: Base note

This evergreen tree comes from Australia and the East Indies. In India the Sandalwood tree is widely considered to be sacred.

Properties
- Antiseptic
- Antidepressant
- Antispasmodic
- Anti-inflammatory
- Diuretic
- Calming
- Astringent

Contra-indications
Do not use for depressed people as it may lower their mood even more.

Extraction
Steam distillation of the wood.

Uses
- Bronchitis
- Urinary infections
- Fatigue

In powdered form, Sandalwood is burned during religious ceremonies.

It helps nervous tension and anxiety either as a blended massage oil or in a vaporiser or burner.

Added to a bath or massaged on the lower back as a blended oil it may help alleviate cystitis.

Sandalwood helps to improve the immune system.

Massaged into the chest or throat as a blend it helps sore throats and bronchitis.

Sandalwood is widely used in beauty preparations and has a beneficial effect on eczema, acne and dry and chapped skin.

Scent
Sweet, woody, warm.

Combines with:
- Frankincense
- Jasmine
- Rose
- Geranium
- Ylang-Ylang

VETIVER (VETIVERIA ZIZANIOIDES)

Effects: Grounding
Aroma: Base note

This is a scented grass native to India and Indonesia. It is from its abundant roots that the oil is produced.

Properties
- Antibacterial
- Anti-fungal
- Calming

Contra-indications
None.

Extraction
Steam distillation of the roots.

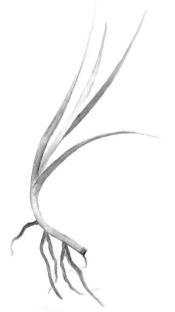

Uses
- Arthritis
- Nervousness
- Insomnia
- Stress
- Mature skins

Vetiver has a very calming effect and is used to treat anxiety and nervous tension.
It is used in the perfume industry.

Scent
Heavy, sweet, woody, earthy.

Combines with:
- Sandalwood
- Geranium
- Lavender
- Ylang-Ylang

GINGER (ZINGIBER OFFICINALE ROSCOE)

Effects: Warming
Aroma: Top note

This plant originates from India, China, Africa and Australia. Ginger root is used extensively in cooking, as it is an excellent digestive aid.

Properties
- Analgesic
- Antidepressant
- Expectorant
- Stimulant
- Digestive aid

Contra-indications
Ginger may irritate sensitive skins.

Extraction
Steam distillation of the dried and ground roots.

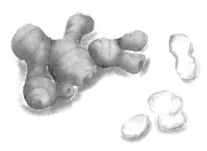

Uses
- Catarrh
- Colds and flu
- Arthritis
- Indigestion
- Constipation

Ginger is also helpful for stimulating poor circulation.
It can be used to ease arthritis, rheumatism and sprains either as a blended massage oil or as a compress.
It is useful in respiratory conditions such as bronchitis, sinusitis etc.
It can be helpful in digestive problems such as flatulence, colic, diarrhoea. It has a positive effect on the nervous system and can help nervous exhaustion.

Scent
Woody, warm spicy.

Combines with:
- Eucalyptus
- Cedarwood
- Citrus oils

Terminology

A guide to descriptions found in the essential oil directory.

Analgesic – this means pain - relieving
(Chamomile, Lavender, Rosemary)

Antidepressant – this lifts the mood
(Bergamot, Geranium)

Antifungal or fungicidal – this inhibits mould and fungi growth
(Lavender, Tea-tree)

Antibiotic – This kills pathogenic bacteria
(Tea-tree)

Antiseptic – this is cleansing and prevents the development of microbes
(Bergamot, Eucalyptus, Lavender, Tea-tree)

Anti-inflammatory – this helps to reduce and prevent inflammation
(Clary Sage, Patchouli, Sandalwood)

Antispasmodic – this relieves muscle spasm in smooth muscle
(Chamomile, Ginger, Lavender)

Antiviral – this destroys certain viruses
(Tea-tree)

Astringent – this contracts blood vessels and body tissue
(Lemon, Sandalwood, Myrrh)

Antibacterial or bactericidal – this inhibits bacteria growth
(Bergamot, Lavender, Lemon, Rosemary, Tea-tree)

Carminative – this reduces intestinal spasm
(Chamomile, Lavender. Peppermint)

Decongestant – this reduces congestion
(Eucalyptus, Rosemary)

Detoxifying – this helps the body to get rid of waste products
(Juniper, Lemon)

Diuretic – this aids urine production
(Cypress, Geranium, Lemon, Patchouli)

Emmenagogue – this encourages menstruation and is therefore not to be used during pregnancy
(Chamomile, Clary Sage, Jasmine, Juniper, Lavender, Marjoram, Rose, Rosemary)

Expectorant – this encourages coughing -up of mucus
(Bergamot, Eucalyptus, Sandalwood)

Fungicide – prevents and combats fungal infection
(Tea-tree, Geranium)

Phototoxic – These oils skin pigmentation on exposure to UV light so must not be used before going in the sun or using sunbeds.
(Bergamot, Lemon, Orange, Grapefruit)

Sedative – this slows down functional activity and lessens excitement, calming
(Chamomile, Clary Sage, Lavender, Rose)

Stimulant – this has an uplifting effect on the body
(Geranium, Peppermint, Rosemary)

Essential Oils

The following are simply guidelines for making oil blends for specific conditions, and as you become more familiar with the oils you will doubtless find that you prefer to make up your own combinations. You will find many different combinations recommended for specific conditions as some oils appeal to one person more than another, and some are more appropriate for particular individuals.

ACNE

This is usually caused by excessive secretion of sebum caused by hormonal stimulation.
Essential Oils
Chamomile, Geranium, Lavender, Frankincense, Tea-tree.
- Add to a carrier oil suitable for face massage and gently massage the face.
- Combine with a skin lotion and apply.
- Apply a toner such as rose flower water. (If the face is inflamed do NOT massage).

ANXIETY

Essential Oils
Bergamot, Cedarwood, Chamomile, Geranium, Lavender, Sandalwood, Ylang-Ylang.
- Add to a carrier oil for massage.
- Add to a bath and soak for up to 15 minutes.

ASTHMA

Essential Oils
Cedarwood, Eucalyptus, Lavender.
- Add a few drops to a bath.
- Combine with a carrier oil for massage. Massaging a few drops of diluted oils on the sternum (breast bone) can help bring relief from the feeling of tightness.
- Do not use inhalations.

ATHLETE'S FOOT

This is caused by a fungal infection.
Essential Oil
Tea-tree.
- Add a few drops to a footbath or dab the area with impregnated cotton wool.

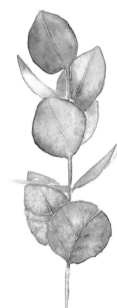

BRONCHITIS

Oils that help bring up mucus will be beneficial.
Essential Oils
Cedarwood, Cypress, Marjoram, Pine.
- Massage the chest and back with the diluted oil.
- Add a few drops in the bath.
- Use as an inhalation.

BURNS AND SUNBURN

Essential Oil
Lavender.
- This can be added to the skin without a carrier oil to treat minor burns.
- Add to a bath.
- Use as a cold compress.

BRUISES

Essential Oil
Lavender.
- Add to a bath.
- Dab the area with 1-2 drops on cotton wool.
- Use as a cold compress.

CATARRH

Essential Oils
Cedarwood, Eucalyptus, Lavender, Lemon, Rosemary, Sandalwood, Tea-tree.
- Add a few drops to the bath.
- Use as an inhalation or compress.

CELLULITE

Essential Oils
Rosemary, Geranium, Lemon, Juniper, Fennel.
- Add to a carrier oil for massage.
- Skin brush regularly with the essential oils.
- Add a few drops of the oils to a bath.

CHILBLAINS

Essential Oils
Rosemary, Lavender, Chamomile, Marjoram.
- Add to a bath or a foot bath.
- Apply as a compress.
- Dab the affected area with the mixed oil.

COLD SORES

Essential Oils
Tea-tree or Eucalyptus.
- Apply 1-2 drops to the affected area with cotton wool.

COLDS

Essential Oils
Eucalyptus, Lavender, Lemon, Marjoram, Pine, Peppermint, Tea-tree.
- Add several drops to the bath.
- Use as an inhalation or in a vaporiser.
- Massage the throat and chest with diluted oils.

CONSTIPATION

The main causes are low roughage, lack of exercise, hurried meals and stress.
Essential Oils
Rosemary, Marjoram, Orange, Black Pepper.
- Add to a carrier oil for massage of the abdomen.
- The use of physillium husks or linseed in the diet is very helpful.

Bran is not recommended as it can irritate the digestive tract. Regular meal times and adequate exercise are also important.

CORNS

Essential Oils
Lemon.
- Dab with a few drops added to cotton wool.

CYSTITIS

This is an infection of the urinary tract.
Essential Oils
Bergamot, Juniper, Lavender, Sandalwood, Tea-tree, Chamomile.
- Add to carrier oil and massage the abdomen and lower back. (If the person has a temperature or is passing blood in the urine they must visit their doctor).
- Add a few drops of the oil to a bath.
- Use as a hot compress on the lower back.

DANDRUFF

Essential Oils
Rosemary, Lavender.
- Use as a hair tonic massaged into the scalp a few times a week.
- To make the tonic add a few drops of each oil to 200 ml of distilled water and 2 teaspoons of cider vinegar in a dark glass bottle. Make sure that you give it a good shake.

EARACHE

Essential Oils
Chamomile, Lavender.
- Use as a compress.

ECZEMA

Essential Oils
Chamomile, Lavender, Sandalwood, Geranium.
- Add a few drops to a bath.
- Combine with a carrier oil and massage gently. (Take care as the skin may be very sensitive).
- The use of Evening Primrose Oil as a supplement or face cream can be beneficial.

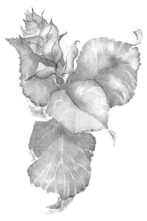

EMOTIONAL STATES

The following can be used as a massage blend or added to a bath.
Depression
Chamomile, geranium, lavender, sandalwood, ylang-ylang.
Insecurity
Sandalwood, frankincense.
Loneliness
Marjoram.
Poor Memory
Rosemary.
Panic Attacks
Lavender, ylang-ylang, frankincense.
Low Self-esteem
Sandalwood, ylang-ylang.

EXHAUSTION AND FATIGUE

Essential oil
Lavender, Geranium, Rosemary.
- Add to a carrier oil for general massage.
- Add to bath water and soak for about 115 minutes.

ACHING FEET

Essential Oil
Peppermint.
- Add to a bowl of warm water and soak feet for 10 minutes.
- Add to a carrier oil for foot massage.

FLATULENCE

Essential Oils
Basil, Fennel, Rosemary.
- Add to a carrier oil and massage the abdomen.

HAEMORRHOIDS

These normally occur due to constipation and can cause great discomfort.
Essential Oils
Cypress, Frankincense.
- Add a few drops to a bath.

HAY FEVER

Essential oil
Juniper.
- Combine with a carrier oil and massage the sinus areas.
- Add a few drops to a tissue and inhale.

HEADACHE

Essential Oils
Chamomile, Rosemary, Lavender, Peppermint.
- Add to a carrier oil and massage around the temples, the base of the skull and anti-clockwise on the solar plexus. Massaging the neck and shoulders can also be helpful as some headaches are caused by tension in these areas.
- If the person is suffering from a migraine headache then massage should not be given.
- Use as a compress or inhalation.
- Add a few drops to a bath.

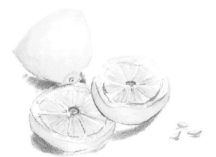

IMMUNE SYSTEM (TO BOOST)
Essential Oils

Lavender, Lemon, Tea-tree.
- Use as an inhalation or in a vaporiser.
- Combine with a carrier oil for massage.
- Add a few drops to the bath.

INDIGESTION
Heartburn and indigestion are very common problems and can be eased by the use of the following oils. If the symptoms last for several weeks then the person should visit their doctor.
Essential Oils

Chamomile, Peppermint, Lemon, Fennel.
- Add to a carrier oil and massage the stomach and anti-clockwise on the solar plexus.
- Drinking chamomile, peppermint or fennel herbal tea is also helpful.

INFLUENZA
Flu is a viral infection which can have unpleasant symptoms such as aching muscles and fever. Fever is a sign of the body trying to rid itself of the problem and should be left to run for up to 48 hours providing it is not too high.
Essential Oils

Lavender, Peppermint, Tea-tree, Marjoram, Lemon, Cypress, Eucalyptus.
- Peppermint oil will help to reduce the problem and ease congestion. (Do not use for babies oryoung children).
- Muscular aches can be eased by baths or rubs using marjoram and lemon which will help eliminate toxins. (Do not massage in cases of high temperature).
- Use as an inhalation.

INSECT BITES
Essential Oils

Lavender, Chamomile, Tea-tree, Lemon.
- Add the oil to two tablespoons of a carrier oil and apply to the affected area. Lavender or Tea-tree oil can be used neat.
- To ease swelling apply a cold compress containing a few drops of chamomile and lavender.
- Add a few drops to a bath.

INSOMNIA
Essential Oil

Chamomile and Lavender.
- Add to a carrier oil and give a relaxing back massage.
- Add a few drops of lavender oil to the bath or one drop to a pillow.

IRRITABLE BOWEL SYNDROME
Essential Oil

Chamomile.
- Add to a carrier oil for an abdomen massage.
- Add a few drops to a bath.

MENOPAUSE SYMPTOMS
Essential Oils

Clary Sage, Geranium and Sandalwood, Lavender.
- Add a few drops to a carrier oil to give a relaxing full body massage.
- Add a few drops of oil to the bath.

MOUTH ULCERS AND GUM INFECTIONS
Essential Oils

1 drop of Tea-tree, Geranium and Lemon added to half a glass of water for use as a gargle.
- Dab the ulcer with 1-2 drops of tea-tree added to cotton wool.

MUSCULAR SPASM
Essential oil

Clary sage.
- Massage the area with the diluted oil.

PAINFUL PERIODS
Essential Oils

Chamomile, Clary Sage, Rosemary.
- Add to a carrier oil and give full body massage.
- Add to a bath or use as a compress.

IRREGULAR PERIODS
Essential Oils

Chamomile, Clary Sage, Geranium, Lavender.
- Add to a carrier oil for massage.
- Add to a bath.

HEAVY PERIODS
Essential oil

Cypress.
- Add to carrier oil for massage.
- Use as a compress or add to a bath.

POSTNATAL DEPRESSION
Essential Oils

Bergamot, Chamomile and Neroli.
- Add to a carrier oil and give a full body massage.
- Add a few drops of oil to a bath.

PREMENSTRUAL SYMPTOMS
Essential Oils

Lavender, Chamomile and Geranium.
- Add to a carrier oil and massage the whole body using relaxing strokes.
- Add a few drops of the oil to a bath.

RHEUMATISM AND ARTHRITIS
Essential Oils

Rosemary, Chamomile, Lavender, Juniper.
- Add to a carrier oil and massage into the affected area.
(Do not massage over any swollen areas or inflamed joints).

- Add 10- 15 drops to a warm bath and soak for 15 minutes.

Rheumatic conditions benefit from cleansing diets containing plenty of fresh fruit and vegetables and grains. Stimulants such as tea and coffee are best avoided.

Arthritis also benefits from diets which help clear toxins from the body. Gentle exercise and keeping the joints warm are also helpful.

SINUSITIS

This can be extremely painful around the top of the nose and across the cheeks. If the problem persists a doctor should be visited.

Essential Oils

Lavender, Eucalyptus and Tea-tree, Peppermint (for inhalations), Rosemary, Bergamot and Juniper (for massage).

- Add to a bowl of hot water and inhale. (Do NOT use this method if an asthma sufferer).
- Using a few drops added to a of carrier oil massage around the base of the skull using circular movements, press on the acupressure points at the base of the nostrils and at the inner corners of the eyebrows and gently work along the eyebrows using a pinching movement.

SKIN CARE

Blackheads

Essential Oils

Pine, Eucalyptus, Lavender

- Use as a facial steam adding the Oils to a bowl of hot water.

Broken capillaries / thread veins

Essential Oils

Chamomile, Neroli, Rose.

- Use combined with facial oil, cream or lotion.

Dry skin

Essential Oils

Chamomile, Sandalwood, Rose, Lavender, Neroli.

- Use combined with facial oil, cream or lotion.

Mature skin

Essential Oils

Frankincense, Geranium. Rose.

- Use combined with facial oil, cream or lotion.

Normal / combination skin

Essential Oils

Chamomile, Lavender, Neroli, Rose.

- Use combined with facial oil, cream or lotion.

Oily Skin

Essential Oils

Cedarwood, Frankincense, Geranium, Bergamot, Ylang-ylang, Lemon, Rosemary.

- Use combined with facial oil, cream or lotion.

Sensitive Skin

Essential Oils

Geranium, Lavender, Rose, Chamomile

- Use combined with facial oil, cream or lotion, but in very weak mixture.

Wrinkles

Essential Oils

Neroli, Frankincense

- Use combined with facial oil, cream or lotion.

SORE THROAT

Essential Oils

Tea Tree,Lavender, Sandalwood, Lemon.

- Add to a carrier oil and gently massage the neck and shoulder area using downward strokes.Massaging the chest can also be helpful.
- A compress can also be used.
- A few drops can be added to a bath.

STRESS

Essential Oils

Sandalwood, Chamomile, Lavender, Clary Sage, Bergamot.

- Add to carrier oil and give a full body massage or if time is limited massage the back, shoulders, neck and face as these areas hold a lot of the tension.
- Add a few drops of the essential oil to the bath.

SPRAINS

Essential Oils

Rosemary, Chamomile and Lavender.

- Add to a carrier oil and gently massage around the effected joint with light strokes, but do not massage swollen areas.
- Apply a cold compress to the swollen area.

TOOTHACHE

Essential Oils

Clove, Peppermint.

- Use as a compress.

VAGINAL THRUSH

Essential Oils

Bergamot, Rose and Lavender or Tea-tree oil.

- Add to a carrier oil and massage the abdomen and lower back.
- Add several drops of oil to a bath.

VERRUCAE AND WARTS

Essential Oils

Lemon, or Tea-tree.

- Dab the affected area with neat oil.

ROOM DISINFECTANT

Essential Oils

Eucalyptus, Lavender, Lemon.

- Use in an oil burner.

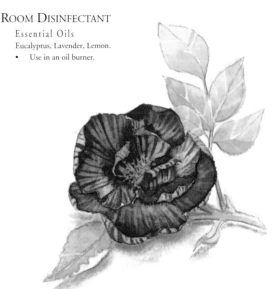

methods of
Extraction

There are a variety of ways that essential oils can be extracted, although some of these are less commonly used today. The most common method currently in use is steam distillation, although there are various more efficient and economical processes being developed all the time.

Steam Distillation

The plant material is placed into a still which is similar to a very large pressure cooker. Steam under pressure is passed through the plant material. The heat causes the globules of oil in the plant to burst open and the oil will evaporate quickly.

The essential oil vapour and the steam then pass out of the top of the still into a water-cooled pipe. The vapours are condensed back to liquids and the essential oil separates from the water and floats to the top. These oils must be stored in dark-coloured bottles in a cool place as they are adversely affected by heat, oxygen, light and moisture.

If stored under the correct conditions, as described, oils should last quite some time. However citrus oils such as lemon and orange are best kept for about six months only.

Some essential oils, notably rose and jasmine, are very expensive due to the fact that the petals of these flowers produce quite a low yield. It has been estimated that more than eight million jasmine flowers are required to produce one kilogram (2.2 lb) of jasmine oil.

Maceration

This process produces what is known as an 'infused oil' rather than an essential oil. Plant material is soaked in a vegetable oil, heated and strained. The oil mixture can be used for massage.

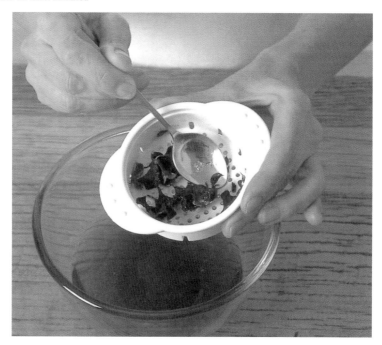

Maceration is a good method for extracting oils for massage purposes.

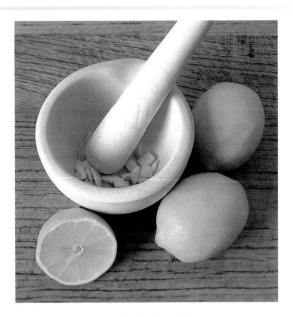

Before cold pressing, rinds are chopped and ground.

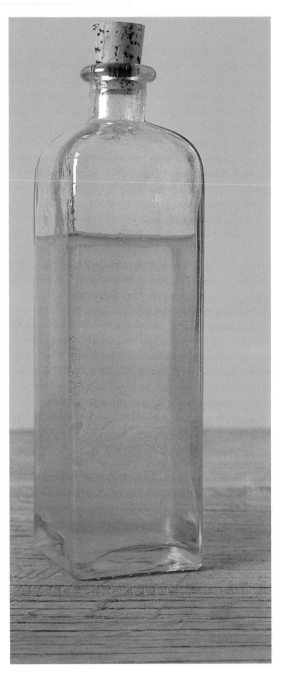

Enfleurage

This method uses wooden frames with a plate glass top which are covered with warm lard. Flower petals are spread over the layer of grease and replaced at regular intervals until the lard is saturated with the essence. Alcohol is then used to wash the grease away and obtain the essence. Any remaining lard can be used in soap making. Although this method is useful for essences which tend to disappear in the process of distillation it is used very rarely these days.

Cold Pressing

This process is used for obtaining essential oils from citrus rinds such as orange, lemon, grapefruit and bergamot. The rinds are ground or chopped and then pressed. The resulting liquid is a mixture of essential oil and watery components which, if left, will separate. In the past the rinds were squeezed into sponges. Oils produced by cold pressing have a relatively short shelf life.

Oils should be stored in a cool, dark place.

Solvent Extraction

A hydrocarbon solvent is added to a drum containing plant material to help dissolve the essential oil. The solution is then filtered and concentrated by distillation and we are left with a substance containing resin known as a resinoid or a combination of wax and essential oil known as concrete. The oil is finally obtained by a process of extraction using pure alcohol.

The alcohol then evaporates and the residual solution is called absolute. Oils produced by this method are not ideal as the solvents are toxic substances and there is always a small residue left behind in the oil which could cause allergies and affect the immune system. Rose and jasmine are extracted by this method.

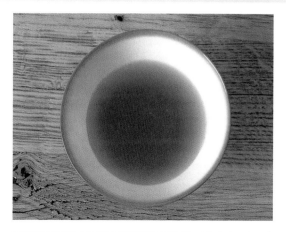

Carbon Dioxide

This is a recently developed method. Carbon Dioxide or butane, can extract the essential oil from the plant when liquefied under pressure. The resulting liquid is drained and allowed to depressurize and the carbon dioxide returns to a gas. The pure essential oil remains.

The same plant can sometimes be treated by different methods to obtain different oils. For example, orange essence is produced from the skins of oranges by the method of cold pressing, while neroli essential oil is produced from the orange blossom by solvent extraction.

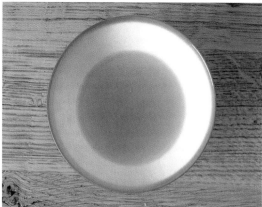

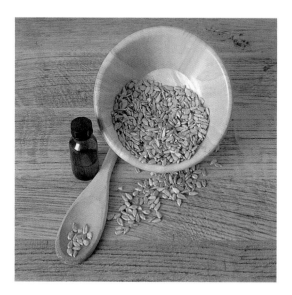

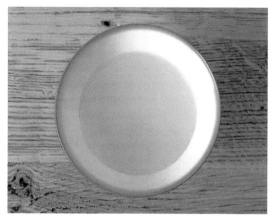

Oil can also be extracted from different plants, fruit and seeds for use as a carrier oil.

The different extraction methods and various parts of the plant used will produce varying strengths of each essential oil.

methods of aromatherapy
Application

A few drops of essential oils can be added to bath water to help relaxation and improve the skin. The essential oil should be mixed with a little carrier oil before adding to the bath and then stirred well. This is a particularly enjoyable way to relax whilst benefiting from these wonderful oils.

The oils can be used as an inhalation by adding about 2-3 drops to a bowl of almost boiling water and inhaling for around 10 minutes to ease blocked sinuses, chest complaints and colds. (This method is NOT to be used by asthma or allergy sufferers). Facial steaming with essential oils is often used in beauty treatments for deep cleansing and moisturising of the skin.

Gargles and Mouthwashes

These are an excellent way of dealing with throat infections, mouth ulcers and gum problems. Add two drops of the oil to a glass of water and use as a mouthwash.

Herbal Teas

These teas are an excellent way of taking herbs and plants internally to improve bodily functions. However they should be used in moderation as they do have medicinal properties. In some countries such as France, doctors give essential oils by mouth but this could have certain dangers as the oils are very potent and is NOT to be recommended unless administered by a medically qualified practitioner. Herbs can also be used in cooking.

Compresses

These can be hot or cold and are prepared by adding 2-5 drops of the oil or oils to a bowl of water. A flannel is used to skim the top of the water and applied to the affected area for about 15 minutes. If hot and cold compresses are used alternately, hot should be applied first, followed by the cold compress. Compresses are ideal for treating swollen joints, backache and headache.

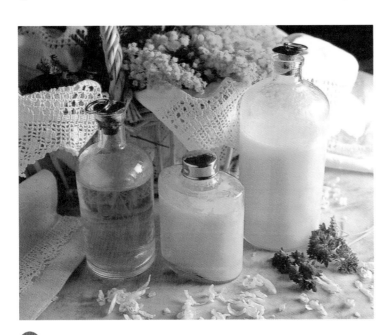

A few drops of essential oil can be added to bath oils and creams to enhance relaxation.

Room Sprays

A clean plant spray is filled with water and a few drops of essential oil added. Shake well and spray in the room. Lavender is ideal for this purpose.

Vaporisation

With this method a few drops of oil are added to a bowl of water which is placed over a small candle. Special oil burners are widely available and make attractive ornaments. The essential oil gradually evaporates into the room. Care should be taken to ensure that the water does not boil dry. This is an ideal way of scenting a room.

Foot Bath

This is wonderful way to relax after a tiring day and is ideal for easing aching feet. Simply add a few drops of essential oil to a bowl of hot water and soak the feet. Peppermint oil is particularly good for this.

Skin and Hair Care

Essential oils can be used as skin moisturisers when added to a carrier oil such as Jojoba.

You can also add them to fragrance-free and lanolin-free creams or lotions to create your own skin care products.

Essential oils can also improve the condition of your hair as well treating as scalp disorders. A few drops of essential oil added to a jug of warm water can be used as a final hair rinse. Chamomile is excellent for fair hair while rosemary is recommended for darker hair.

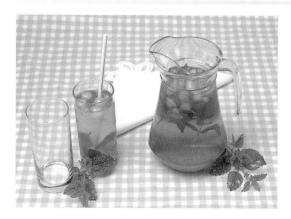

Herbal teas can be helpful, but should only be used in moderation.

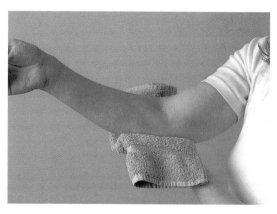

A hot or cold compress can ease swollen or aching joints.

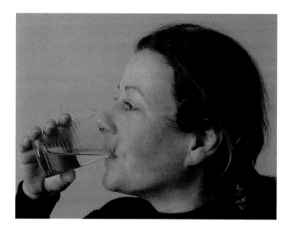

A couple of drops of oil in a glass of water makes an effective mouthwash.

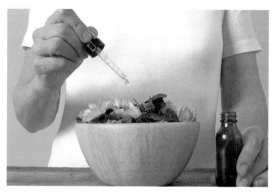

Another way to scent a room is to add a few drops of your favourite oil to a pot pourri mixture.

buying and storing Oils

It is very important to select pure, natural and good quality oils for use in Aromatherapy. In an ideal situation the use of oils produced from organically grown plants would be the first choice. However in reality oils from organic plants are not always easy to obtain and can be costly.

The price of the oil will give you a good indication of its quality. It is always recommended that you avoid buying cheap, poor quality oils, as these may cause allergic reactions.

The oils should always be stored in dark coloured bottles and the neck of the bottle should contain a dispenser so that one drop can be obtained at a time.

Always use a reputable specialist supplier, and be prepared to ask if the oils are pure and where they have come from. As you become more familiar with the essences you will be able to tell if the oil is fresh and has its characteristic odour.

It is better to buy undiluted oils and mix them yourself with a carrier oil. The oils keep better this way and this will give you more flexibility.

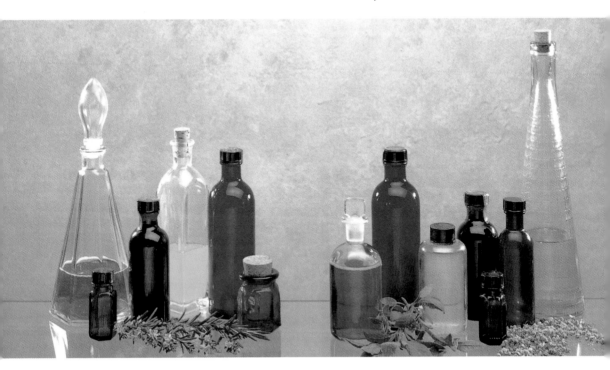

To keep oils for as long as possible, always store them correctly.

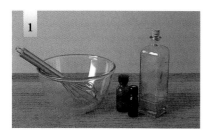

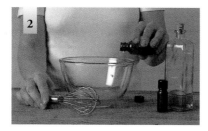

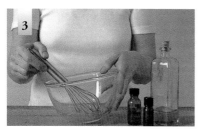

Mixing up your own oils is a relatively easy process.

Store oils in dark-coloured glass bottles. Do not mix up too much at any one time.

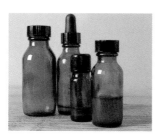

Essential oils are concentrated and fairly expensive, and when using them in an Aromatherapy treatment you would normally mix them with a carrier oil. There are numerous vegetable oils which can be used as carrier oils, the most commonly used being olive oil, grapeseed, almond, sunflower, wheatgerm and avocado.

To dilute an essential oil you need a clean, empty glass bottle of about 50ml (around 2 fl oz) capacity which you can obtain from most chemists. To this bottle you should first add your carrier oil and then your essential oil. (A small plastic funnel will be helpful for decanting the carrier oil).

You can choose one essential oil or use a mixture of several, but the total number of drops of essential oil will be about 20-25. It is best not to use more than three essential oils in a blend. Gently shake the bottle to ensure that the oils have mixed together and make sure that you label and date the contents. Adding about 25ml (about 1 fl oz) of wheatgerm will help to preserve your mixture should you wish to keep it for future use.

For 30ml (1 fl oz) of carrier oil add 12-15 drops of essential oil.
For 20 ml (1/2 fl oz) of carrier oil add 8-10 drops of essential oil.

For people with sensitive skin and children up to twelve years old, a weaker mixture can be made up using 50 ml (around 2 fl oz) of carrier oil and 12 drops of essential oil.

The percentage concentration of the essential oil in the mixture should be between 1-3%, but it is now considered to be more appropriate to use the lower concentration.

It is advisable not to mix large quantities as the blended oils can quickly turn rancid. The mixed oils should be stored in a cool, dark place and should keep for up to three months.

Do not store essential oils in plastic containers as the oils may react with the plastic causing the container to deteriorate which will affect the properties of the oils.

carrier
Oils

The importance of diluting essential oil with a vegetable carrier has been explained, and some of the most popular carrier oils are described below. Vegetable oils do not keep for long so it is important to keep them in a cool, dark place. Always use pure, cold-pressed vegetable oils.

GENERAL-USE CARRIER OILS

Sunflower Oil

This is an ideal oil for general purposes as it contains essential fatty acids and is rich in vitamin E. It is golden yellow in colour and has a slightly nutty smell.

Almond Oil (sweet)

This is a very soothing oil and is easily absorbed by the skin. It contains vitamin D and has beneficial effects on hair, dry skin and brittle nails. Almond trees are abundant in the Mediterranean region and the oil is extracted from the kernel.

For a richer blend it can be mixed with jojoba or avocado oils.

Grapeseed Oil

This oil is extracted from grape pips. It is one of the least expensive oils, and is good for oily skins. It has a light texture and can be mixed with almond or avocado oils for use in massage.

Soya Oil

This comes from the soya bean plant and is easily absorbed. It is rich in vitamin E.

Specialist Carrier Oils

These can be added to the general carrier oils for specific purposes such as nourishing and soothing dry skin.

Avocado Oil

This is extracted from the flesh of the avocado, and is ideal for dry, ageing and sensitive skins. It contains vitamins A and D and has a rich texture.

Jojoba Oil

This contains a high level of waxy substances which mimic the

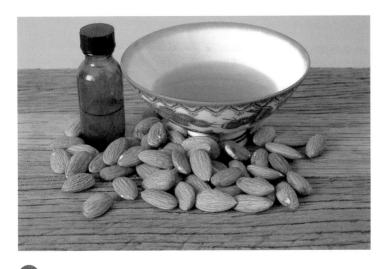

Almond Oil

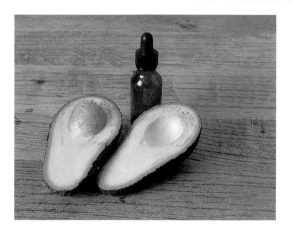

Avocado Oil

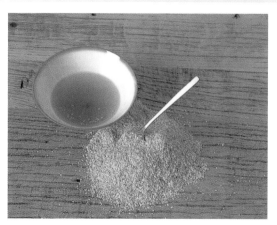

Wheatgerm Oil

skin's own collagen, helping to keep it supple. It is ideal for the face and is beneficial for spots and acne. It is rich in vitamin E, helps to condition hair and can be used to treat dandruff and a dry scalp.

Wheatgerm Oil
This contains vitamins A, B, C and E and helps to alleviate blemishes as well as firming and toning the skin. It has a rich texture and can help reduce scar tissue and stretch marks. It does, however, have quite a strong smell and is best used combined with other oils. It can also be added to general carrier oil blends to help prolong their life.

Apricot Kernel
This helps to keep the skin smooth and is rich in mineral salts and vitamin A.

Peach Kernel
As the name implies, this oil is extracted from the peach kernel and contains vitamins A and E as well as essential fatty acids. It is very beneficial for the face and can be combined with almond or grapeseed for a richer blend.

Evening Primrose Oil
This oil, extracted from the seeds of the plant, is helpful for skin conditions such as eczema and psoriasis. It can be blended with jojoba oil but only keeps for about two months after opening.

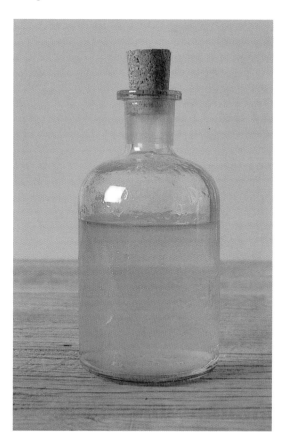

Carrier oils can be stored for mixing with your essential oils.

the effects and benefits
of Massage

Massage is possibly the oldest healing art in the world. Ancient manuscripts from India, China and Egypt refer to massage and Greek and Roman physicians used massage for pain relief and healing.

Massage not only benefits the receiver but also the giver. We are being massaged all the time without being aware. For example, when we breathe the diaphragm – the large muscle between the abdomen and chest – moves up and down, massaging our internal organs. This form of massage is essential to our daily lives.

Just the touch of a hand can be very reassuring to a baby who has hurt themselves or a sick person or someone who is simply feeling a little lonely and isolated. Massage can be considered to be a holistic form of therapy as it works on all levels, bringing harmony to mind, body and spirit. If the body is calmed and relaxed then the mind will also feel less anxious.

Today massage is an important therapy throughout the world. When we consider the many ways in which it can help the body this universal popularity is not surprising.

PHYSIOLOGICAL BENEFITS OF MASSAGE

Circulation
During massage, the amount of blood pumped to the heart is increased, which affecs blood pressure. Local arterial, capillary and venous flows are improved.

Massage expands capillaries, causing a temporary reduction in systolic and diastolic blood pressure and a small increase in the heart rate. Urine flow is increased and cellular metabolism is also improved.

Joints
Pain in the joints can be due to injury, inflammation or simply wear and tear. Massage can be beneficial in reducing the pain and speeding up the healing process.

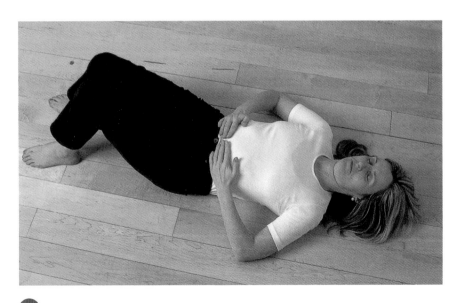

Correct breathing techniques are important as they effectively massage our internal organs.

Lungs

Massaging the chest, shoulders and back can not only help to reduce tension but can also greatly improve breathing. As massage also assists the removal of congestion from the lungs, respiratory conditions can also be alleviated.

Skin

During a massage, sweat may be increased which helps the removal of toxins from the body.

Nervous system

Our nervous system helps regulate all other systems of the body, so by calming the nerves with massage we are indirectly helping all the organs of the body to operates more effectively.

Digestive System

Stress, long working hours and irregular meals can wreak havoc with our digestive system. Symptoms such as bloating, indigestion and constipation are only too common these days. Massage can have a profound effect in improving the functions of the digestive system by helping to ease indigestion and flatulence. It can also be beneficial in cases of constipation.

Lymphatic System

This is the system of the body which helps fight infection, so it is very important that it is kept in good working order. Massage helps release congestion in the lymphatic system, which in turn helps to improve our immune system.

Muscles

We all know the problems that tension in the muscles can cause, particularly in the neck and shoulders. Massage helps ease spasms and tension, enabling taut muscles to work efficiently once more. It can be very beneficial both before and after sport to keep muscles in good shape and to help prevent damage.

Emotions

Pent-up emotions can often lead to tension in the muscles so by relaxing the muscles, massage also helps to release any unexpressed emotions.

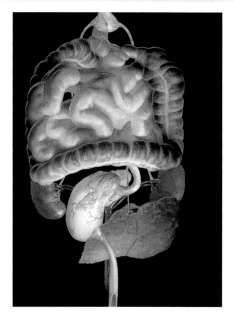

Many parts of the body can be adversely affected by stress, particularly the digestive system.

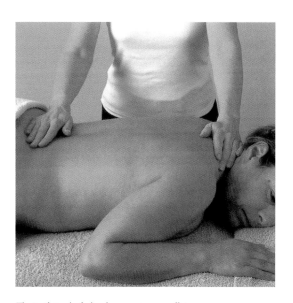

The simple touch of a hand can ease stress or suffering

Preliminaries

The aim of an Aromatherapy massage is to make the person feel peaceful and relaxed. With this in mind, it is therefore important to create a warm, friendly atmosphere with soothing lighting and minimal noise – soft music can often be enjoyable.

The Room

The room should provide a warm, comfortable setting with a calming, relaxing atmosphere. Temperature is also important, as if your partner feels too cold, they will not be able to relax properly. Similarly, if the room is too hot, relaxation will also be impossible. A room temperature of around 25° is ideal.

Your aim is to keep noise to a minimum, so use a room away from street or traffic noise, and avoid interruptions. Unplug the telephone and make sure that any other people around will not disturb you for the duration of the massage.

Massage Surface

Of primary importance is the receiver's comfort, so the massage should be given on a firm, but padded, surface. Purpose-built couches can be bought or hired, although the floor is perfectly suitable as long as it is adequately cushioned. However, beds are not ideal massage surfaces. Generally the height of a standard bed is not suitable for massage purpposes, and most beds are rarely firm enough to allow the application of the correct pressure.

A purpose-built couch has the advantage of placing less strain on your back and legs. If using a massage couch, make sure that the height is correct. To check positioning, stand with your arms straight at your sides. If the palms of your hands can rest easily on the top of the couch, then the position is correct.

At least when you begin, it is likely that you will be practising your massage using the floor. This has some advantages in that you can use any room, and the person being massaged has plenty of room to spread out. If the floor is to be used it should be covered with a couple of blankets or a piece of foam rubber.

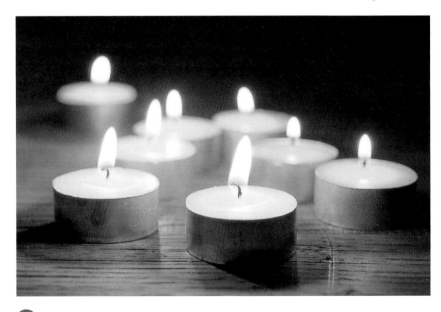

Candles can help create a soothing atmosphere.

Small cushions can be placed under the receiver's neck and the back of their knees for added support and comfort. It is also important for you to kneel on a soft surface to protect your knees. If you have any problems with your knees or back it is advisable that you use a massage couch.

The person being massaged should always be kept warm so it is important to have a good supply of clean, warm towels available for this purpose. Always start each massage by placing a clean, warm towel on the massage surface for the receiver to lie on, and also cover him/her with a warm towel, as this will make them feel more relaxed. Throughout the massage, only the area of the body being worked on should be uncovered.

Clothes

When giving a massage it is important to wear loose comfortable clothing, although they should not be so loose that they get in your way. Shoes should be flat and light or if you prefer, you can go barefoot. Do not wear any jewellery as this may scratch the receiver's skin, as well as being a distraction or irritation for you. You should always wash your hands before and after the massage.

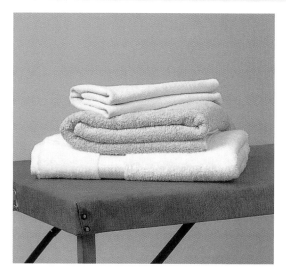

Always make sure you have a supply of fresh, clean towels to hand.

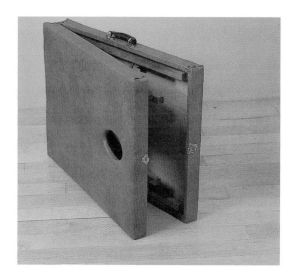

A purpose-built couch is ideal for massage, although not essential.

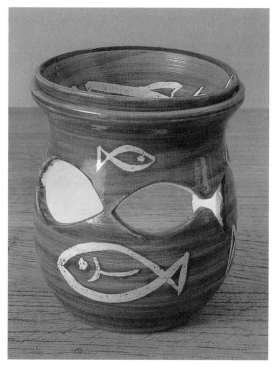

A few drops of a favourite oil in a special burner will enhance relaxation.

Giving a massage can be quite tiring so it is important to try and keep as relaxed as possible. If you are feeling tense or suffering from a cold or flu then it is best not to give a massage.

Finger nails should be kept as short as possible to avoid causing any unnecessary discomfort to your partner. Hands and nails should also be scrupulously clean and should be washed immediately before starting a treatment and as soon as the treatment is finished.

It is also important to make sure your hands are warm before touching the receiver's skin as cold hands could make them tense.

Always add the oil to the palms of your hands before applying it to the body and try to keep one hand in touch with your partner's body throughout the massage sequence to maintain the flow.

Timing a Massage

To give a full body massage you need to allow at least one hour. If time is limited, rather than rushing, it is preferable to concentrate on a particular area such as the back or head and face. These are particularly good areas for easing stress and tension and generally take about 20 minutes.

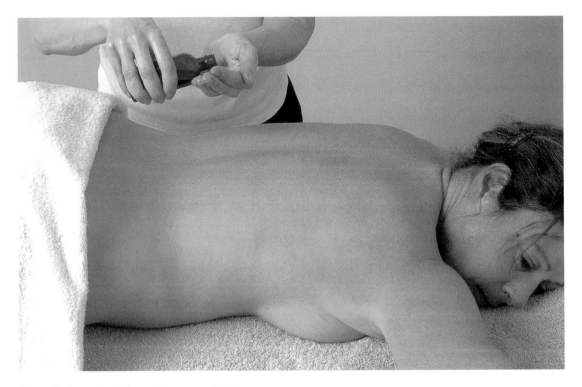

Always add oil to your hands before touching your partner's body.

Hands can be kept supple using the following exercises:

1. Put the palms of the hands together then lift your elbows so that your palms no longer touch. Press the fingers together as tightly as possible and hold for six seconds (1-2).

2. Hold a small rubber ball in one hand and repeatedly squeeze and relax you fingers around it (3). Repeat with other hand.

When giving the massage, your back should be kept straight and the weight of your body used to give rhythm and depth to the massage. If working at a couch, stand with your feet apart and bend your kneel leaning into the strokes. If working on the floor, kneel with your knees apart. Do not stay in one position for too long and always face the direction of the massage strokes.

The pressure of the strokes should be varied to add interest and variety, remembering that some people will prefer firmer strokes to others so it is a good idea to ask for feedback as the person being massaged will know best what feels right for them. Light strokes are preferable over bony areas and firmer strokes over large muscles such as the buttocks.

Try to relax as much as possible and use flowing strokes. Do not worry about following sequences too rigidly. It is better to simply go with the flow. The more happy and relaxed you are, the more the receiver will enjoy their massage experience.

It is advisable not to talk too much during the massage as you need to concentrate on what you are doing and your partner needs to be able to relax and let go of any tension, whether mental or physical.

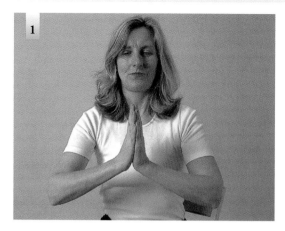

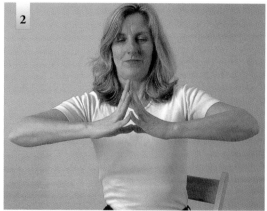

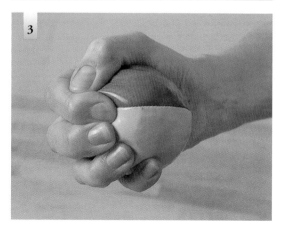

contra-indications for
Massage

Although massage is of enormous benefit there are a few occasions when it should not be given.

Never massage someone with the following conditions without their doctors permission.

- Heart condition
- Recent serious operation
- Open wounds or burns
- Viral or bacterial infection such as flu
- Cancer
- Inflammatory conditions such as thrombosis
- Acute back pain
- Pregnancy

It is important to remember that massage stimulates the flow of blood and lymph and can easily spread infection around the body.

Do Not Massage:

- over varicose veins.
- swollen or painful rheumatic joints.
- fractured bones.
- over lumps or tumours.
- immediately before or during menstruation. Care should be taken as the increased flow of blood could make the period very heavy.
- over the abdomen in cases of hernia or diarrhoea.
- before the 12th week of pregnancy and only then with their GP's permission.

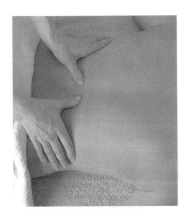
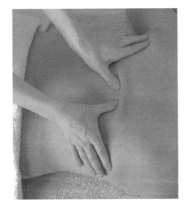
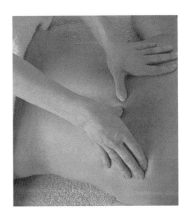

The massage sequences that you will be using in the body massage are made up of just a few basic strokes. These are based on traditional Swedish massage developed by Per Henrik Ling in the 19th century and are known as stroking or effleurage, kneading or petrissage, percussion or tapotement and friction.

Although they may seem a little complicated to start with, in time they will become easier. It is a good idea to practice on yourself before trying it on friends or family.

STROKING OR EFFLEURAGE

This is very important and versatile and is essentially a stroking movement. It should always be done in the direction of the heart. It can be performed using the palm of the hand, the base of the hands or fingers and thumbs. If practised lightly it works on the surface tissues while firmer pressure acts on deeper tissues. It is generally used at the beginning and end of treatments and as a connecting movement between other strokes. It is also used to spread massage oil over the body.

You can do a full body massage with effleurage alone by varying the depth and rhythm of the strokes. For a good general back massage, stroke with a sweeping motion up the back, beginning at the base of the spine (1), up to the shoulders (2.3) then fanning out and down along the sides (4,5,6).

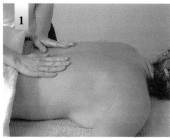

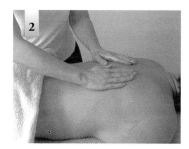

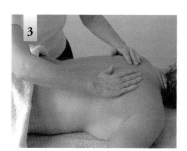

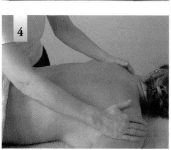

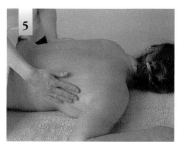

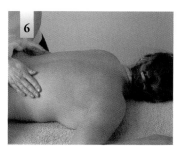

CIRCULAR STROKING

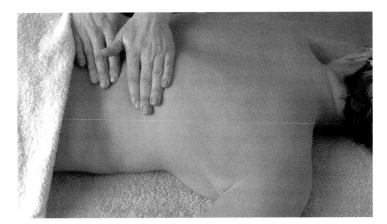

This is performed with the palms of the hands. Simply stroke around the area in a circular motion, repeating as many times as you wish.

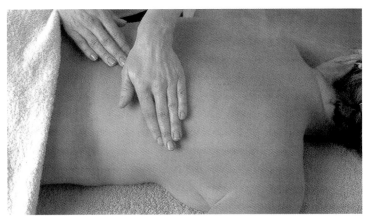

This stroking movement should be done very softly, so as not to irritate the receiver's skin.

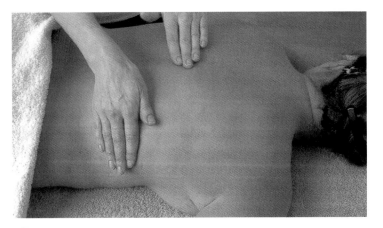

Continue with this stroke covering the whole area. Repeat as desired.

FEATHERING

This is a wonderfully calming stroke and is an ideal way to finish a back massage. Starting at the shoulders stroke very lightly down the back with one hand and then the other.

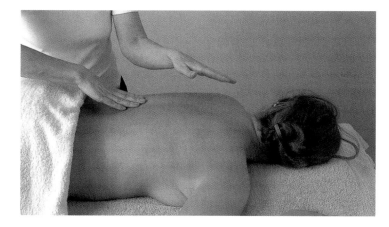

As the name of the stroke implies, your touch should be feather-light. Your hands and arms should be very relaxed and the stroke very smooth.

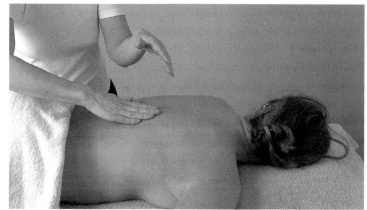

As with circular stroking, continue this technique as long as you wish.

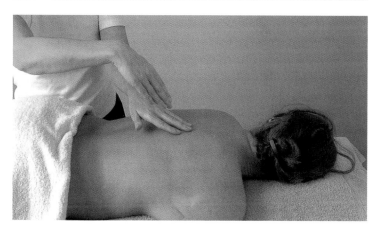

KNEADING OR PETRISSAGE

This movement is like kneading dough and follows venous circulation. This can be performed with one hand or both hands. The muscle is lifted from its base between the thumb and fingers and then squeezed along the muscle fibre.

This stroke stretches and relaxes tense muscles, improves circulation and helps the absorption and elimination of waste products. It is useful on the shoulders and the fleshy areas such as the hips and thighs.

Light pressure kneading will work on the surface muscles and the skin. To work on the deeper muscles a firmer movement will be required.

It is advisable to combine the kneading with petrissage as it is hard work and can be tiring for you and the receiver.

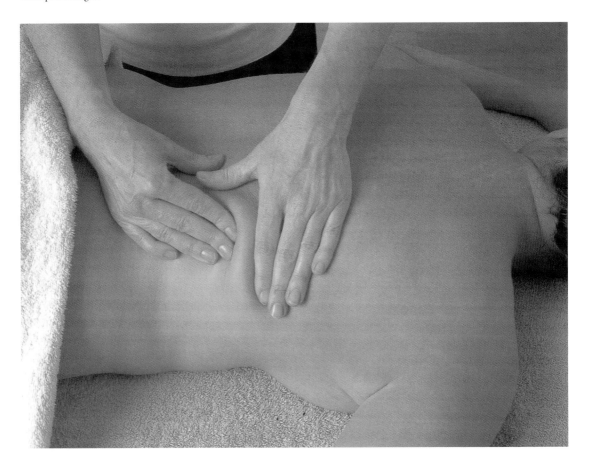

FRICTION

Strictly speaking this could come under the heading of effleurage, as it could be considered to be a stroking movement but it is generally classed as a separate technique.

This movement is carried out with the thumb pads pressed down hard on the skin. With progressive tiny circular movements of the thumb, move over the surface being treated in a series of straight lines along the muscle. It is important to press on the underlying tissues so that the skin is moved with the pressure.

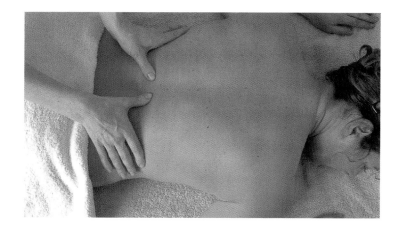

Static friction can also be used by applying pressure with the pads of the thumbs. This is often done on either side of the spine. The fists can be used for strong muscles.

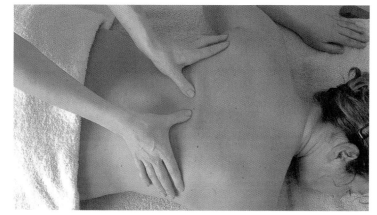

This is a good technique for breaking down rheumatic or fatty nodules and is most effective on areas where the muscle lies over a bony surface such as the area over the scapula. It also relieves pain and relaxes muscles.

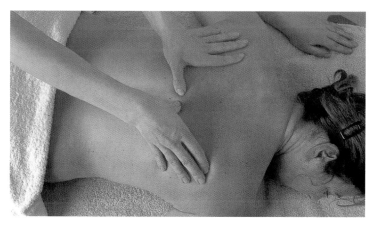

PERCUSSION OR TAPOTEMENT

There are a number of variations that can be described under this heading. Each improves circulation and is generally stimulating. This technique is best used on fleshy muscular areas such as the buttocks and thighs.

HACKING

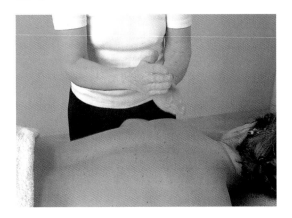
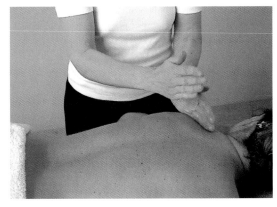

This is done by 'hacking' or tapping the skin. Strike the skin with the sides of your hands, flicking them away just as you touch the skin. Use your hands alternately and work very quickly.

Keep the movements light and springy with relaxed wrists and fingers and never use them on bony areas or over broken veins and bruises.

CUPPING

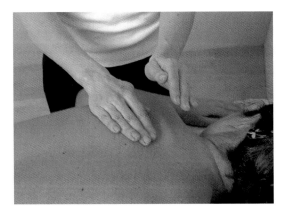
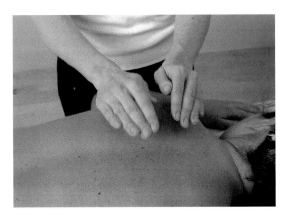

This is another version of percussion, and is performed with fingers together and slightly bent to form a cup shape. Air between the hands and the body creates a softer stroke. When the movement is performed correctly you will hear a plopping sound.

The movement is made by striking the skin with alternate cupped hands. Cupping is most effective on the back to relieve congestion and mucus in respiratory conditions.

PUMMELLING

This can be performed with clenched fists, using alternate hands as you would for hacking. Simply strike the skin with the fleshy part of your fists.

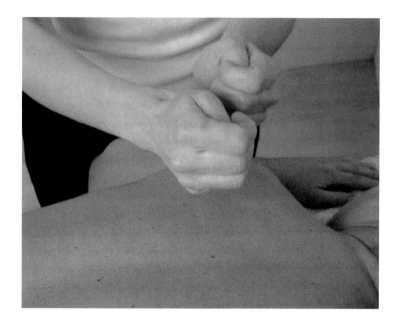

PLUCKING

As the name implies, here you pluck small amounts of flesh between your thumbs and fingertips. Do be careful not to pinch the skin.

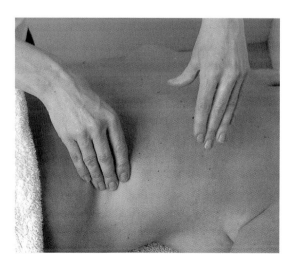
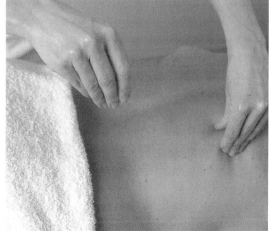

facial
Massage

This can be incorporated into the body massage sequence after the head, neck and shoulders and before the hand, or it can be used as a very relaxing massage in its own right.

Massaging the face can release a great deal of tension, and is excellent for helping to relieve headaches. The improved circulation to the area also gives the person a look of glowing health and vitality.

It is important that the receiver removes any contact lens before having a facial massage. You will need to use a face oil or face cream for this massage.

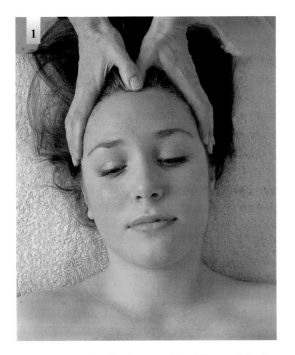 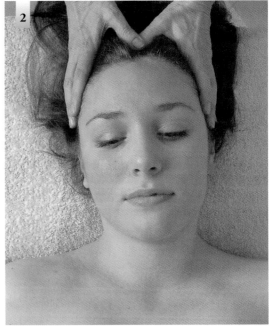

STEP 1. Stand or kneel at the receiver's head. Do not oil hands at this stage. Starting at the top of the forehead in the centre place one thumb on top of the other. (1) Then press at one inch intervals, moving from the centre of the forehead up over the top the head to the back of the head and down towards the back of the neck as far as you can reach. (2) Repeat this movement several times.

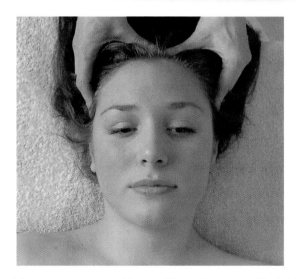

STEP 2. Spread the fingers of each hand out over the top of the skull and firmly massage all over the head. Make sure that you massage firmly enough to move the skull.

(If the receiver does not like their head being touched, simply omit steps two and three, and progress straight to step four).

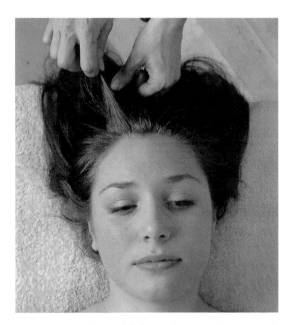

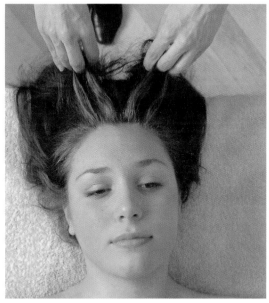

STEP 3. Grasp a clump of the hair at the roots and pull it, gently but firmly.

Release and let your fingers run through the hair. Using alternate hands, work over the scalp.

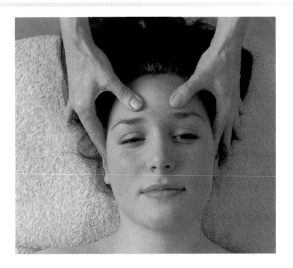

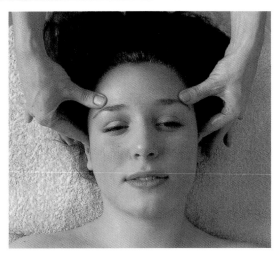

STEP 4. Apply the facial oil to the palm of your hands and gently apply it all over the face and neck area. Stand or kneel at the head and place the balls of your thumbs side by side in the centre of the receiver's forehead just below the hairline.

Stroke the thumbs latterly in opposite directions out towards the temples where thumbs should break contact and return to the centre of the forehead. Repeat the movement, moving slightly further down the forehead each time until the whole forehead has been covered.

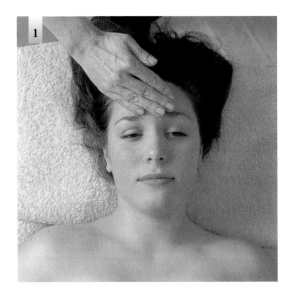

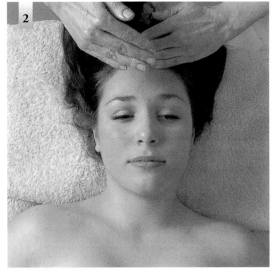

STEP 5. Place the palms of your hands horizontally across the forehead. One hand should be above the other. Using a rolling motion, brush one hand over the forehead, followed by the other

hand. Start at the right hand side of the forehead and work out across towards the left and then return to the right. Repeat several times. (Sequence 1-2)

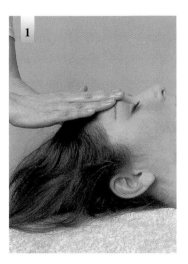

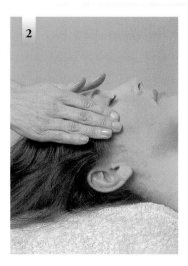

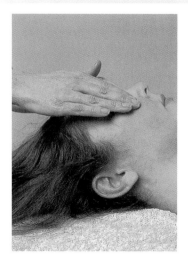

STEP 6. Place your hands either side of the bridge of the nose, fingers pointing downwards, finger tips touching the eyebrows. Stroke out along the eyebrows with the finger tips. Circle on the temples and glide back under the eyes to the nose. Repeat twice. (Sequence 1-2)

Then place the palms of your hands carefully over the receiver's eyes and hold for a few seconds before lifting them away very slowly.

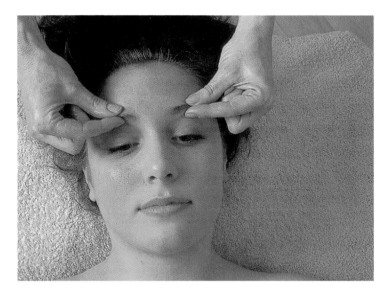

STEP 7. Using the thumb and first finger of each hand, firmly pinch the bone above the eye, working outwards from the nose. Repeat this movement several times

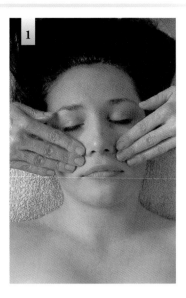

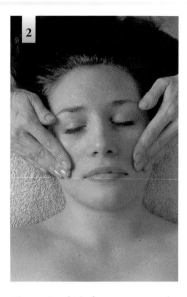

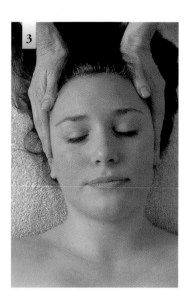

STEP 8. Place the fingers of each hand either side of the nose, pointing inwards over the cheeks (1).

Then, using fairly firm pressure, stroke the fingers over the cheek and out to the ears. Repeat several times. (2-3)

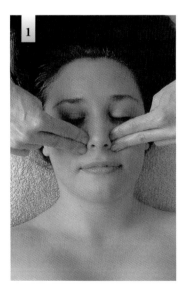

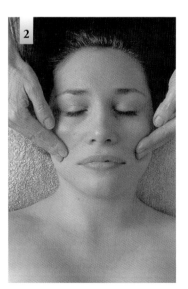

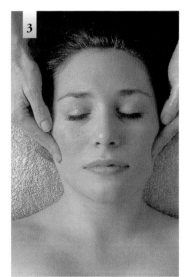

STEP 9. Using the first two fingers of each hand, place them at the sides of the base of each nostril. (1)

Then press inwards, hold for a count of ten and then sweep the fingers of each hand out to the ear. (2,3)

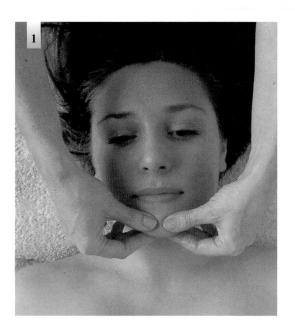

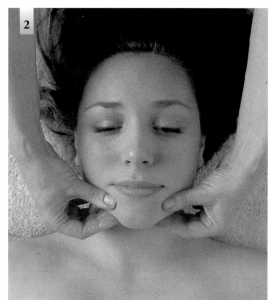

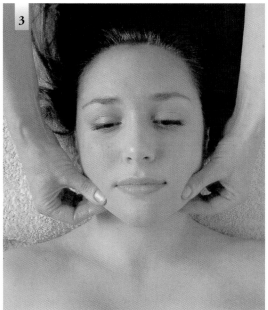

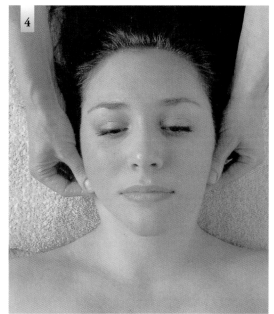

STEP 10. Place the thumbs at the centre of the jaw bone with your fingers underneath the jaw bone. Beginning at the centre, make little circles with your thumb on the jaw bone out towards the ear. Repeat this several times. (1-4)

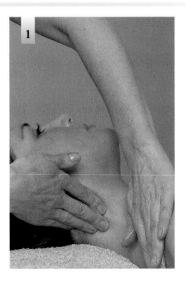
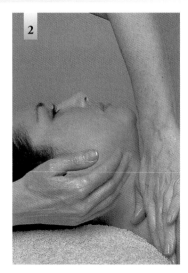
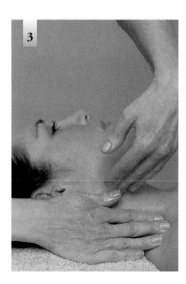

STEP 11. With the palms of your hands stroke up the neck from the shoulder to the ear using first one hand and then the other on both sides of the neck. Repeat several times.(Sequence 1-3)

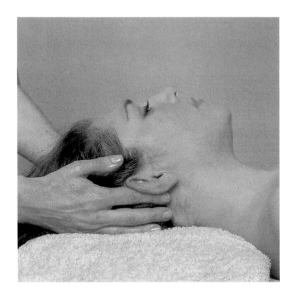
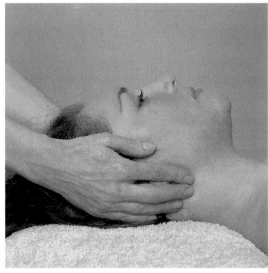

STEP 12. Place the tips of your fingers behind the receiver's ear and stroke up and down the backs of the ears with your finger tips several times.

Place the palms of your hands over the ears and hold for a few seconds before lifting them away very slowly.

body massage

Sequence

Having covered the important massage preliminaries, we are now ready to start the actual massage sequence. There are no set rules as to which part of the body you should start with, but the back is always a good place as the nerves from the spine branch out to all areas of the body. It is also one of the main areas of the body where we carry a lot of tension and the muscles in the shoulders particularly can become tight and knotted.

The sequences described are only guidelines. With practice you will develop your own techniques. And remember that the more you relax and enjoy the massage, the better it will be for both you and your recipient.

BACK MASSAGE

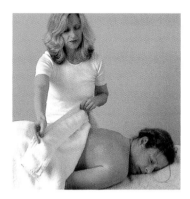

Before you begin the massage sequence, the receiver should be covered with a warm, clean towel. Position yourself to the side either kneeling or standing. Try to relax and concentrate on the massage. Only then pull back the towel to begin.

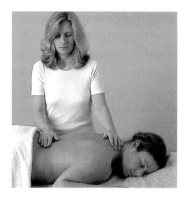

STEP 1   Commence by placing one hand just below the neck and the other at the base of the spine, breathing slowly to help you relax. Hold your hands in this position for a few seconds. This helps both you and your receiver to relax and tune into each other.

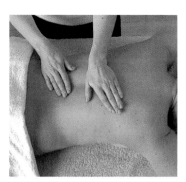

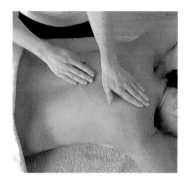

STEP 2   Slowly move the palms of your hands over the receiver's back using slow circular movements. This is like a warm-up before the massage really starts.

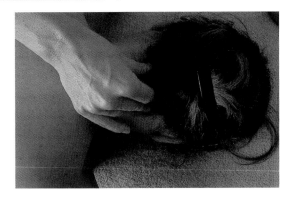

STEP 3 Next start to massage the base of the skull. Using your right hand place the right thumb on the left side of the base of the skull and the fingers on the right side. Pull the thumb and the fingers together. Using the thumbs of both hands, start in the centre at the base of the skull and work out from the centre towards the ears. Press the thumbs along the base of the skull. When you reach the ear return to the centre and repeat several time.

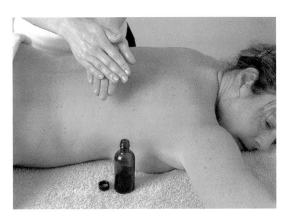

Now add the mixed essential oil to the palms of your hands.

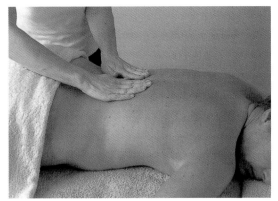

STEP 4 Now place your right hand on the right of the receiver's lower spine and your left hand on the left of their lower spine, fingers pointing towards the spine.

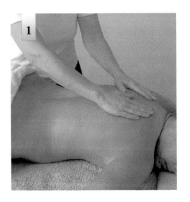

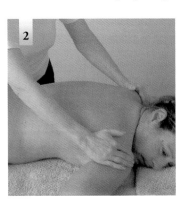

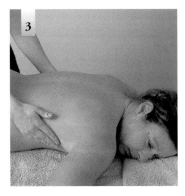

Stroke your palms towards the receiver's neck where they should fan out across the shoulders and the top of the arms, then glide them down the sides of the body. When you reach the waist pull upwards and inwards and then repeat the whole sequence several times. (1-3)

STEP 5 Place the palm of your left hand over the back of your right hand and commencing at the lower back work in a figure of eight movement using effleurage strokes over the whole back. (1-2)

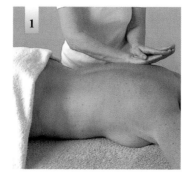
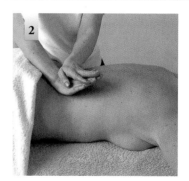

STEP 6 Place the palm of one of your hands on the receiver's shoulder, and the other hand on their lower back on the same side. Slide hands up and down the back, working both hands at the same time in opposite directions. Work up and down across the whole back, but avoiding the spine, several times. (3-4)

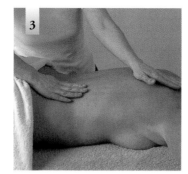
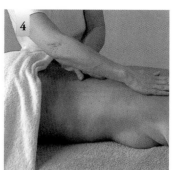

STEP 7 Place the palm of one hand on the lower left hand side of the receiver's back and your other hand on their upper back, with your fingers pointing across the back in the same direction. (5)

Move your hands from side to side across the back, working both hands at the same time in opposite directions. Cover the whole back up to the shoulder area repeating several times. (6)

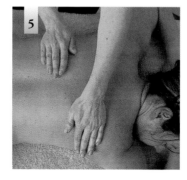
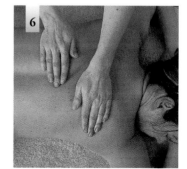

STEP 8 Starting at the base of the spine, place your thumbs either side of the spine. Press firmly and then release the pressure, moving the thumbs a little further up the spine. Repeat the pressure. Continue up the spine to the neck in this way and then return to the base and repeat.

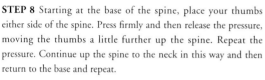
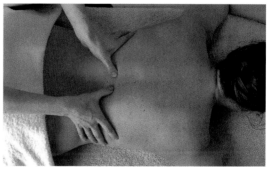

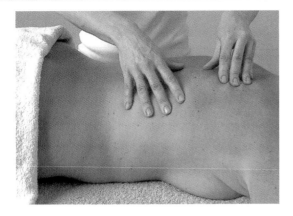

STEP 9 Using the fingers of each hand spread out, work all over the back in circular movements, keeping your fingers straight at all times.

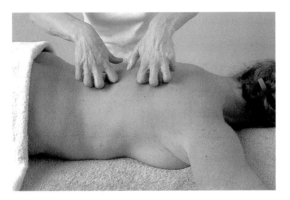

STEP 10 Bend the fingers of each hand and massage over the whole back with the first knuckle joints using circular movements.

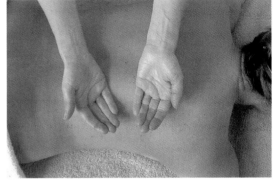

Turn your clenched fists over and massage the back with the backs of your fists, again using circular movements.

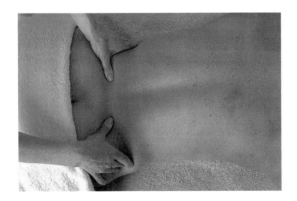

STEP 11 Place your thumbs together above the buttocks in the centre of the back at the base of the tail bone. Making small circles with the thumbs, move out towards the hips and down towards

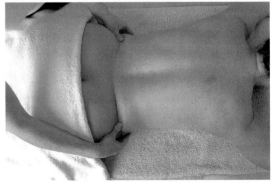

the floor or the couch. Return the thumbs to the centre of the back and repeat the whole sequence again.

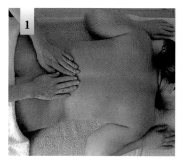
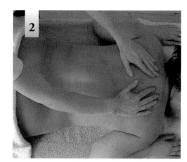
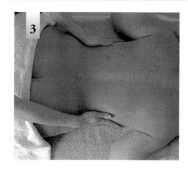

STEP 12 Place your hands at the top of the buttocks, fingers pointing upward, and stroke upward and outward. Then mould them around the sides of the waist and pull firmly up at the sides. Return hands to the starting position and repeat. (1-3)

STEP 13 You are now going to use the kneading movement on the back. Start just above the buttocks and work up the back to the shoulders. Stand or kneel at the side of the receiver and using the palms of both hands alternately, scoop up the skin and roll it between your fingers as you turn your hands inward. Do be careful not to pinch the skin. Work on both sides of the back up to the base of the neck and out towards the top of the arms.

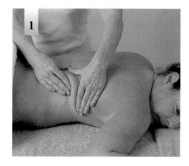
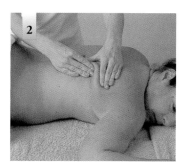

STEP 14 With the receiver's arms flat on the couch, elbows out to the sides and hands above their head, knead the muscles of the neck.

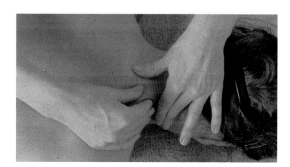

STEP 15 You will now work on the shoulder area using friction. With the balls of your thumbs, work across the shoulder. This can sometimes be quite painful so do take care not to over-work on these areas. Just do a little at a time and follow each friction session with soothing effleurage strokes.

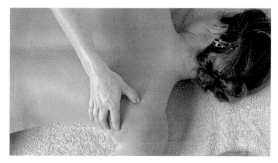

STEP 16 Using your fists for the pummelling movement, start at the buttocks and work your way up the back. Avoid the kidneys at the back of the waist. Your strokes can be firm over the fleshy parts such as the buttock but should be gentler over bony areas. Avoid the spine altogether. Make sure that your wrists are relaxed and the movement is light. It is a good idea to practice these strokes on your thigh before attempting them on others.

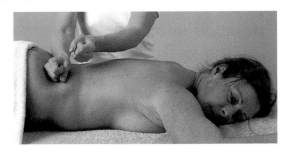

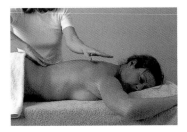

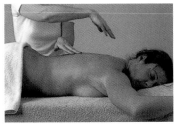

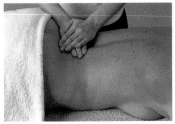

STEP 17 Finish the back massage with a very light stroking movement known as feathering. Beginning at the neck, stroke gently down the spine using one hand at a time.

When one hand reaches the bottom of the spine, the other should be starting at the top. On reaching the small of the back, return your hand to the neck. These stroking movements should gradually become slower and lighter.

Finally place your cupped hands over the small of the back. Gently flatten your hands into the back and lift your hands away very slowly. Now cover the back with the towel.

BACK OF LEG MASSAGE

Leg massage can be of great benefit to those whose jobs require them to stand for long hours as well as being beneficial before and after exercise. It helps to improve the blood supply to the area and can help prevent varicose veins. If however there are varicose veins present then massage in these areas should be avoided.

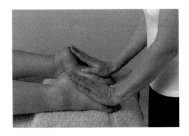

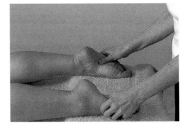

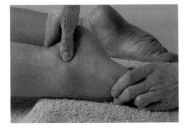

STEP 1 Uncover the feet. Standing or kneeling at the feet of the receiver, place the palms of your hands on the sole of each foot. Keep your hands on your partner's feet for a few seconds then slowly lift them away.

STEP 2 Using your thumb, make circular movements over the soles of the feet, working from the toes towards the heels.

Now work around the ankles with circular movements.

STEP 3 Now oil your hands. Standing beside the receiver's right foot, cup the palms of your hands across the leg close to the heal.

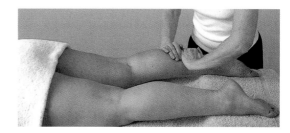

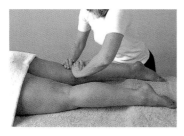

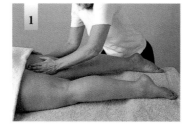

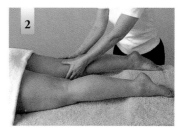

With your right hand above your left hand, stroke up the leg towards the buttocks.

Here the hands should spread out and glide down the side of the leg to return to the heel. (1-2)

STEP 4 Knead the calf muscles using both hands. This whole sequence should be repeated several times. When making stroking movements, your knees should be bent and you should lean into the stroke. Pressure should be gentle over the back of the knee.

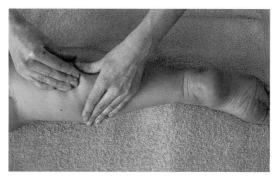

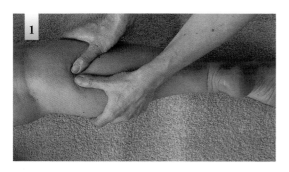

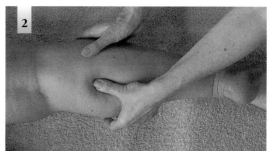

STEP 5 Stroke up the calf with your thumbs. Using alternate thumbs make small upward strokes. Press firmly as you stroke up and out, then more gently as you glide back to the centre. (1-2)

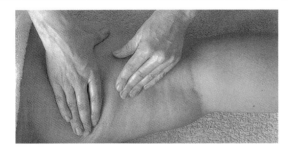

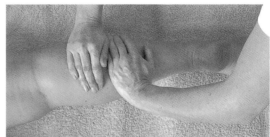

Now continue stroking up the leg to the thigh.

STEP 6 Finish the leg massage by gently stroking the whole leg. Now repeat the whole sequence for the other leg.

The receiver should now be asked to turn over as you are now ready to work on the front of the body. Hold the towel by the corners and lift it up a little so that they can turn over discreetly.

Always stand close to the couch so that they do not roll off. Cushions or pillows can be placed under the head and knees for extra comfort and support.

SHOULDER, CHEST AND NECK MASSAGE

With the receiver lying on their back; stand at or kneel at their head. Uncover the chest area. In the case of a female ensure that only the top of the chest is uncovered and the breasts are still covered with the towel.

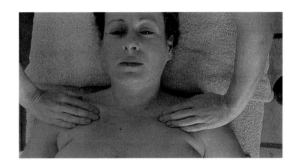

STEP 1 Oil the palms of your hands and start over the collar bones at the top of the shoulders, arms facing horizontal towards each other and the hands about four inches apart. Press down for a count of two.

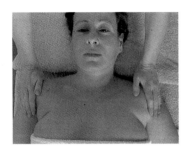

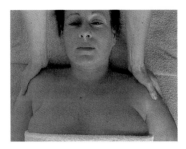

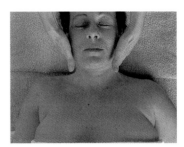

Move hands over the top of the shoulders and press down for a count of two.

Then slide the hands around the back of the shoulders.

Finish by stroking up the sides of the neck.

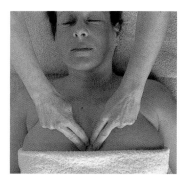

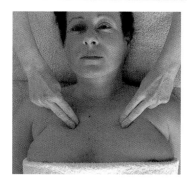

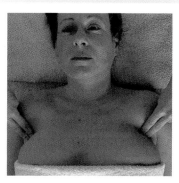

STEP 2 Standing at the head, place the finger tips of both hands at the top of the sternum.

Using circular movements massage up to the collar bones. Massage under the collar bones with finger tips.

Then sweep fingers down towards the armpits. Repeat several times.

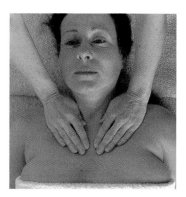

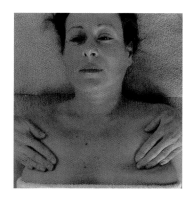

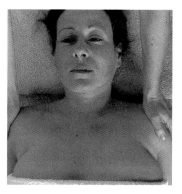

STEP 3 Place hands next to each other just below the collar bones, fingers pointing down.

Stroke down the chest to the top of the breast area. Fan the hands out across the chest towards the shoulders.

Cup your hands over the shoulders. Now swivel your hands around to the back.

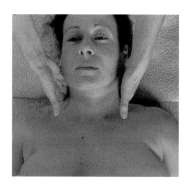

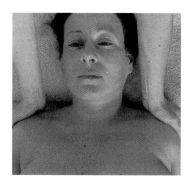

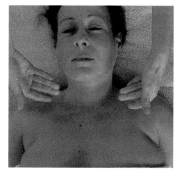

Stroke up the back of the neck.

Then slide the hands around the back of the shoulders.

Then stroke down the sides of the neck to the collar bone. Repeat several times.

STEP 4 Place your hands either side of the receiver's neck. Using stroking movements, massage from the top of the arms up to the base of the skull. Keep the strokes smooth and very gently let the head move from side to side with the strokes.

Finish by gently holding the sides of the head in your palms for a few seconds.

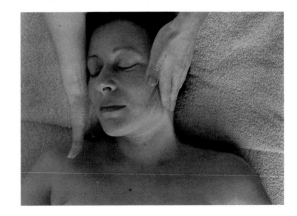

HAND MASSAGE

Hand massage can be comforting and relaxing. With the receiver still lying on their back, stand or kneel by their left arm.

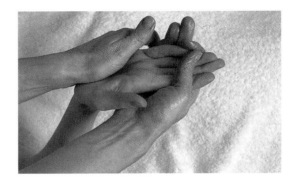

STEP 1 Oil the palms of your hands and hold the receiver's left hand in one of your hands, palm upwards. Stroke their palm with the heel of your hand.

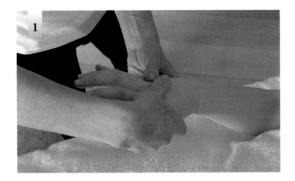

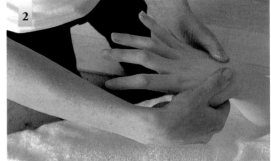

STEP 2 Support the receiver's hand, palm downwards, with your fingers across the palm. Stroke the back of their hand with your thumbs. Stroke out from the knuckles to the wrist. (1-2)

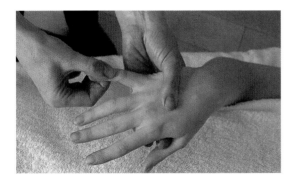

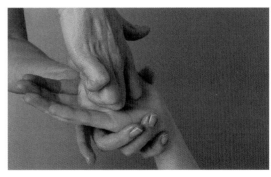

STEP 3 Support the receiver's hand in one of your hands. With your other hand massage each finger in turn starting with the little finger. When you reach the thumb, swap your hands over to make the thumb massage easier. Make sure that you give a thorough massage all around the thumb.

STEP 4 Hold the back of the receiver's hand in one of your hands and massage their palm using your knuckles.

STEP 5 Support the receiver's hands with your fingers and stroke all around the wrist with your thumbs. Work from the centre of the wrist upwards, and then out towards the sides of the arm. (1)

Turn the hand over and work on the other side of the wrist in the same way. (2)

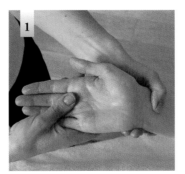

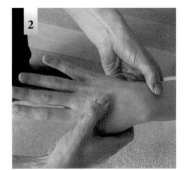

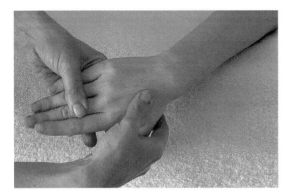

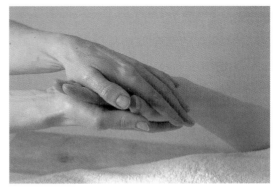

STEP 6 Hold the receiver's hand with both of your hands, thumbs over the top. Stroke between the tendons moving towards the wrist. Use your thumbs one after the other and massage along each tendon a few times.

STEP 7 Finally, stroke their hand between the palms of your hands and on the final stroke slide your hands off the end of the fingers very slowly.

ARM MASSAGE

Although the arms themselves may not seem to be a very important area, many of the problems found in the shoulder and neck area can be closely related to tension in the arms. Many people have jobs that require them to move their hands and arms in a repetitive manner so this area should not be ignored.

With the receiver lying on their back, stand or kneel by their left side. Uncover their left arm only and oil your hands.

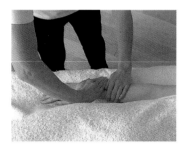

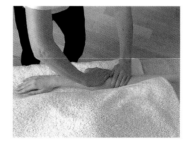

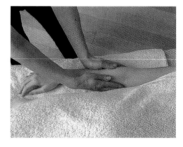

STEP 1 the receiver's arm should be flat on the couch, palm downwards. Place your hands across their wrist, with left hand above your right.

Stroke firmly up the arm towards the shoulder. On reaching the top of the arm, spread your hands out around the shoulder.

Then slide your hands down the sides of arm and return to the wrist. Repeat the sequence several times.

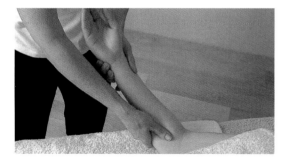

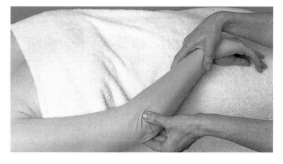

STEP 2 Support the arm at the wrist with one hand and with your other hand stroke up from the elbow towards the wrist using your thumbs. Work on the front and back of the arm.

STEP 3 Support the arm just above the elbow with your left hand, and with the tips of your right fingers or thumb, massage all around the elbow with circular movements.

STEP 4 Gently knead the receiver's lower arm from the wrist to the elbow. Repeat this several times making sure that both sides of the arm are thoroughly covered.

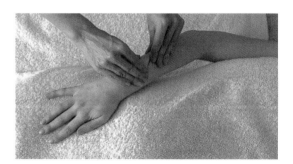

STEP 5 Continue the kneading on the upper arm working from the elbow to the shoulder. Repeat several times.

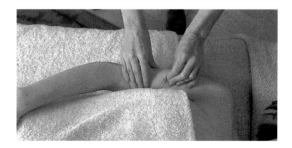

STEP 6 Lift the arm up in the air. Stroke down the arm from the wrist to the shoulder making sure you cover the back and front of the arm. It may be easier to change hands half way through.

Cover this arm. Repeat hand and arm massage for the other arm.

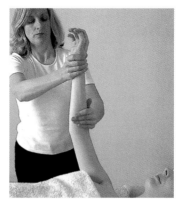

ABDOMEN MASSAGE

This area is very beneficial for easing digestive problems which are often related to tension and anxiety. It is important to keep the strokes gentle.

Uncover the abdomen area and, if massaging a female, place a small towel over the breast area.

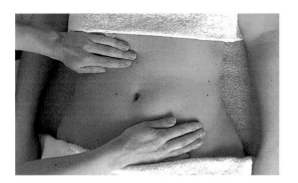

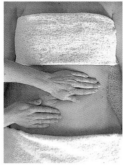

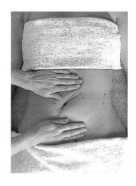

STEP 1 Oil the palms of your hands and standing to the side of the receiver, place your right hand on the right side of the receiver's abdomen just below the rib cage. Your left hand should be palm downwards, on the left side of the receiver's abdomen just above the groin.

Draw the right hand towards you and move over the abdomen, circling the navel in a clockwise direction.

As you start moving your right hand, your left hand should start to move to the right side of the abdomen.

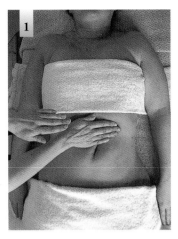

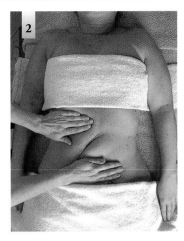

Here it should break contact and return to repeat the movement again when the right hand commences its next cycle. Repeat several times.(1-2)

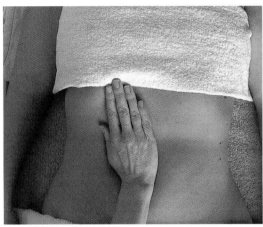

STEP 2 Place the palm of your right hand on the centre of the diaphragm. Gently rock the right hand back and forward several times.

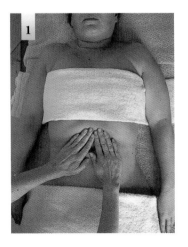

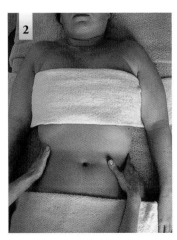

STEP 3 Facing towards the receiver's head, place your hands side by side on the lower abdomen. (1)

Stroke up to the ribs where your hands should fan out across the top of the abdomen to the waist. (2)

Here your hands should be pulled up and inwards and then returned to the starting position at the lower abdomen. Repeat several times.

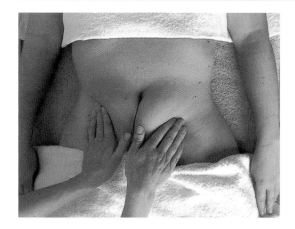

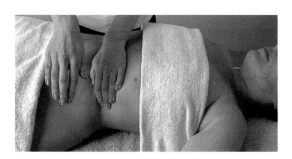

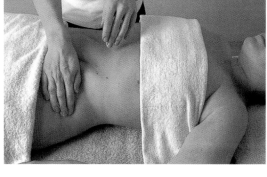

STEP 4 Standing or kneeling at the receiver's side, gently stroke up the sides of the waist with one hand at a time. Keep the strokes

flowing and lift the hand away when you reach the navel. Repeat on the other side.

STEP 5 To finish, cup your hands over the navel. Hold for a few seconds and thenslowly lift them away.

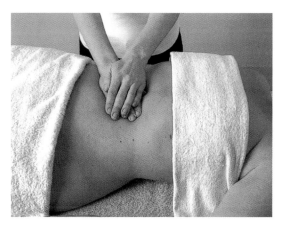

FOOT MASSAGE

Foot massage can be one of the most beneficial treatments for the whole body as the soles of the feet contain many nerve endings which relate to organs all over the body.

With the receiver lying on their back, stand or kneel at their feet and uncover one foot at a time. Keep the legs covered with the towel. Start by massaging the left foot.

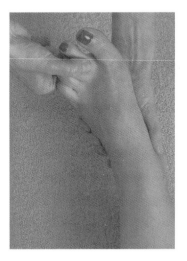
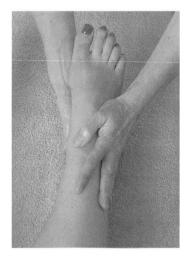
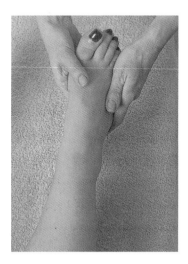

STEP 1 Stroke the foot from the toes towards the ankle by placing your right palm over the top of the foot and your left palm under the sole of the foot. When you reach the ankle, swing the hands round and return to the toes. Repeat several times.

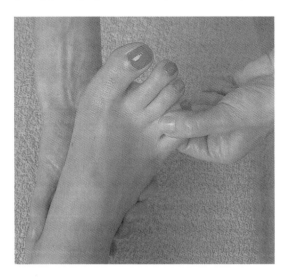
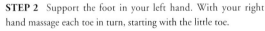
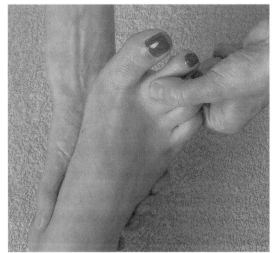

STEP 2 Support the foot in your left hand. With your right hand massage each toe in turn, starting with the little toe.

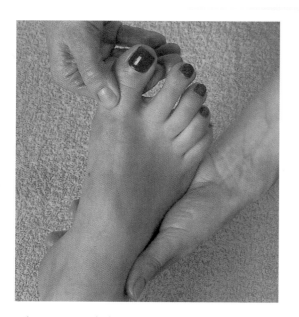

When you get to the big toe, swap hands as this will make the massage easier.

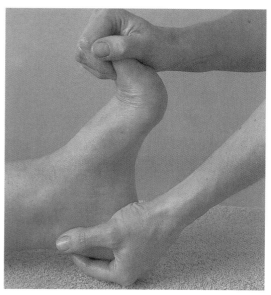

STEP 3 Support the ankle in one hand and clasp the toes in the other hand. Very gently bend them backwards and forwards.

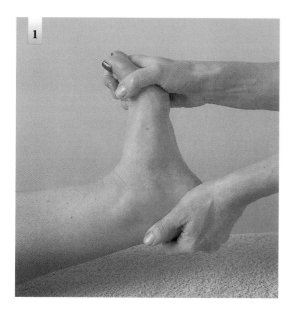

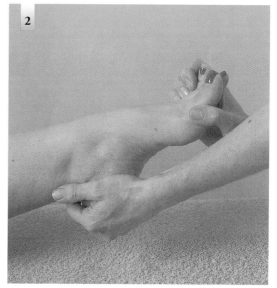

Support the foot at the ankle with one hand and with the other hold the foot across the toes. Flex foot up and down. (1-2)

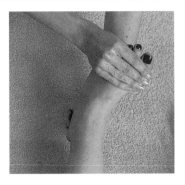
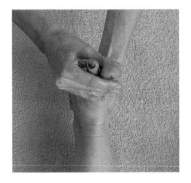
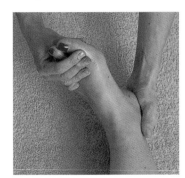

Then turn the foot from side to side, and finally rotate in each direction.

STEP 4 Supporting the foot with your hands, use your thumbs to work over the back and sole, making small circular movements. (1)

STEP 5 Using first one thumb and then the other, stroke between the tendons, working towards the ankle.(2)

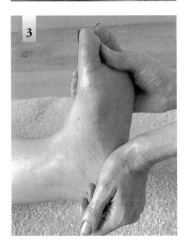
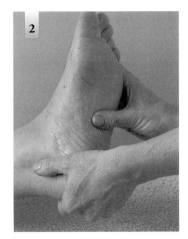

STEP 6 Stroke the sole of the foot with the heel of your hand, moving from the ball towards the heel. (3)

STEP 7 Finish by stroking the receiver's foot between your hands several times. Finally hold the foot for a few seconds before gliding them to the toes very gently. (4)

Repeat steps 1-7 for the other foot.

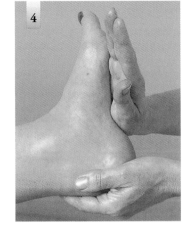

FRONT OF LEG MASSAGE

Stand by the receiver's left foot.

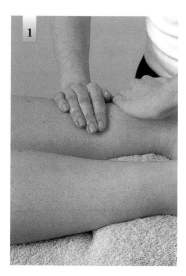
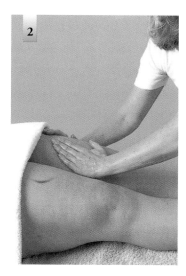
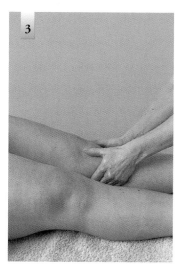

STEP 1 Uncover the left leg and oil hands well. Place your palms across the receiver's left ankle, right hand above your left hand.

Stroke towards the groin, then spread them out and slide them down the side of the legs back to the ankle. (1-3)

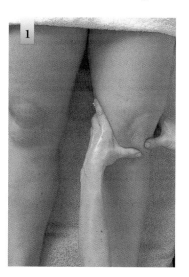
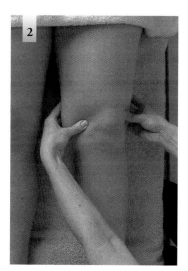
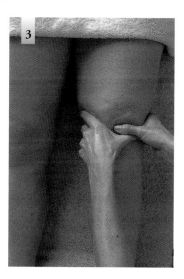

STEP 2 Stroke gently up the side of the knee, one thumb each side, until you reach the top of the knee. Allow the thumbs to pass each other at the top, then glide down the opposite side. Both

thumbs should do a complete circle, passing at the top and bottom of the knee.(1-3). Knead the thigh thoroughly, working firmly on the outer thigh and more gently on the inner thigh.

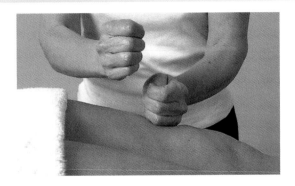

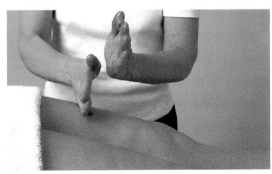

STEP 3 Work on the outside of the thigh, first using pummelling movements.

Now continue using hacking movements.

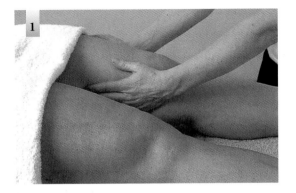

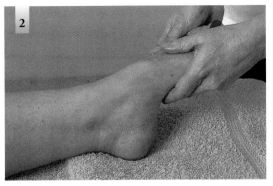

STEP 4 Finish by stroking the leg and on the final stroke slide the hands across the foot and off the end of the toes. (1-2) Cover left leg.

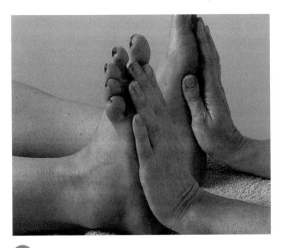

To finish the Aromatherapy massage, place the flat palms of your hands on the soles of the receiver's feet. Hold this for a count of twenty, then very slowly lift your hands away and cover their feet with a towel. Leave the receiver to relax for a few moments. If they have fallen asleep, allow them to wake very gently.

You may like to play relaxing music at this stage, and offer them a herbal tea. At the end of the massage wash your hands and give them a good shake to release any negativity which may have built up.

The massage sequence described is only a guideline and you may wish to develop your own techniques in time. You can change the order in which you work on the different areas but make sure that you do not miss out any of the areas covered when giving a full body massage. Always keep one hand in contact with the body during each sequence.

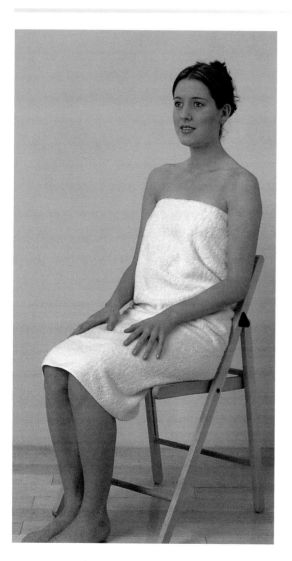

self
Massage

Aromatherapy self-massage, although perhaps not quite as relaxing as being massaged by someone else, will none the less be a very valuable experience.

You will learn more about yourself and the areas which are suffering the most from aches and pains. Self-massage can be done at any time and you can even incorporate it in other forms of relaxation such as watching television.

The strokes that you will use are very similar to those that you have learnt in the previous chapters, so the techniques should come quite easily.

As with all forms of massage, you will benefit most by creating a warm, relaxing atmosphere. Perhaps burning some essential oils and playing soothing music will help add to the success of the session.

Before commencing the massage, it is a good idea to lie on the floor and completely relax all the muscles of the body. (The breathing and relaxation techniques covered in the last chapter could be practised).

Slowly get up and sit in a comfortable position either on a padded floor covering or a comfortable chair. It is important that you choose the position that is right for you otherwise you will be too tense to benefit from the self-massage.

NECK AND SHOULDERS

This is an area where we can all benefit from a release of tension.

STEP 1 Start by massaging the base of the skull. Place your thumbs at the centre of the base of your skull. With your thumbs work out towards your ear. Repeat several times.

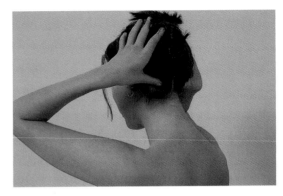

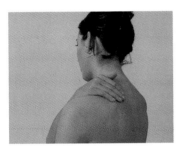

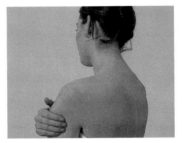

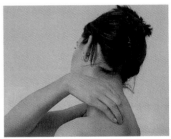

STEP 2 With your right hand knead your left shoulder and work down the top of your arm. Repeat on the other side using your left hand.

STEP 3 With your wrist relaxed, tap your left shoulder with the fingers of your right hand. Repeat on the other side.

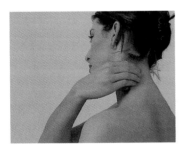

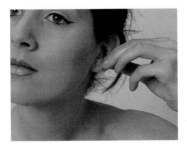

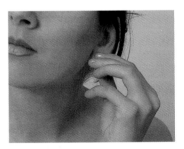

STEP 4 Place the palms of your hands at the sides of your neck just above your shoulders. Using small circular movements, work up your neck towards your ears. Return your palms to the sides of your neck and massage up towards the base of your skull. Work in this way until you reach the centre of the back of your neck.

STEP 5 Using your thumbs and fingers, start to massage your ears beginning at the top and working all the way down to the lobe. Give the lobe a really good massage.

STEP 6 Then taking hold of each lobe in turn between the your thumbs and fingers give them a gentle pull.

FACIAL MASSAGE

STEP 1 Using the palms of your hands, one hand following the other, stroke up your forehead from the top of your nose to your hairline.

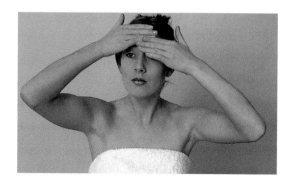

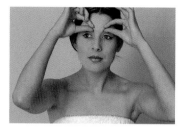

STEP 2 Starting above the top of your nose, pinch along your eyebrows using your thumbs and index fingers.

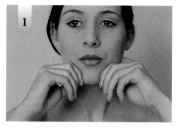

STEP 3 Starting at the centre of your chin, use your thumbs and index fingers to massage your jawbone out towards your ears. (1-2)

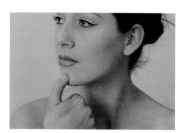

STEP 4 Massage the centre of your chin with the ball of your thumb, making circular movements.

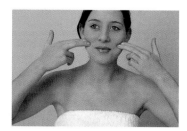

STEP 5 Place your index fingers and middle fingers on each side of your nostrils. Sweep the fingers out under your cheek bones and up towards your ears. Finish by circling on your temples.

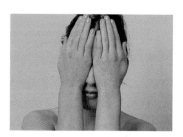

STEP 6 Place the palms of your hands over your eyes. Close your eyes and hold them closed for a few seconds. Press very gently against your eyes, then very slowly lift your hands away.

HAND AND ARM MASSAGE

STEP 1 Take hold of your left hand in your right palm and massage all around your left palm with your right thumb.

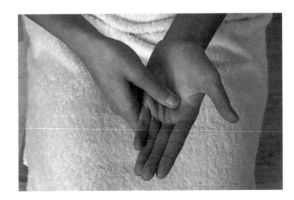

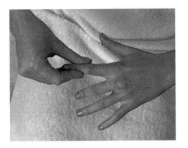

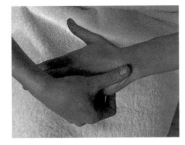

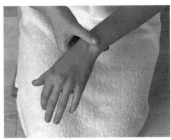

STEP 2 Starting with your little finger, massage each finger in turn including your thumb. Pay particular attention around your joints.

STEP 3 Using your thumb, stroke the back of your hand from your knuckles up towards your wrist.

STEP 4 With your thumb, stroke all around your wrists back and front. Use an upward movement.

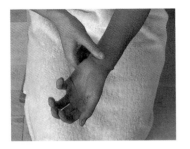

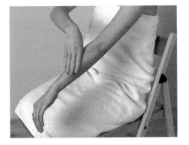

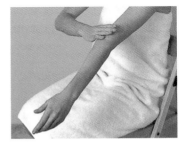

STEP 5 Massage around your elbow, making small circular movements with your fingers.

STEP 6 Stroke up the front of your arm using the palm of your hand from your wrist up to your shoulder.

Mould your palm around your shoulder and massage down the inside of your arm to your wrist.

Repeat the same sequence for your other hand and arm.

ABDOMEN

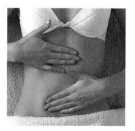 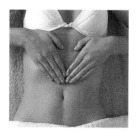 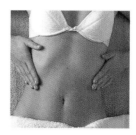 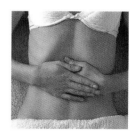

STEP 1 Lying down, place the palms of your hands on your lower abdomen and circle around, one hand following the other.

STEP 2 With the palms of your hands placed side by side at the centre of your lower abdomen, stroke up towards your ribs.

Then fan the hands out to the sides and slide them down the sides of your body.

STEP 3 Place the palms of your hands on top of each other, covering your navel. Hold for a few seconds.

Then gently press before carefully lifting your hands away.

LEG MASSAGE

STEP 1 It is preferable to sit up again for the leg massage. Starting at your ankle, stroke up your leg to your thigh. Use the palms of your hands moulded around the sides of your leg.

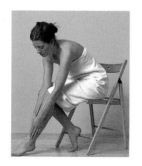

STEP 2 Bend your leg and stroke up the calf muscle. Now place your foot flat on the floor. Gently knead this area and follow with stroking.

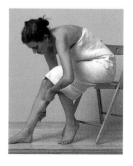

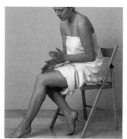 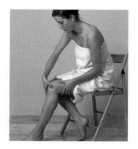 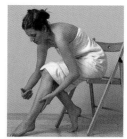

STEP 3 Work on your thighs with kneading movements.

Now use the hacking movement, finishing with some gentle stroking.

STEP 4 With your knee bent, use your thumbs to work around your kneecap.

STEP 5 Finish your leg by stroking up the sides from your ankle to your thigh as in step 1.

FOOT MASSAGE

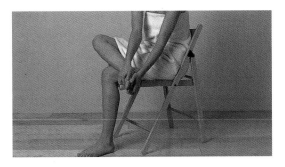

STEP 1 Sitting in a comfortable position, bend your knee over your leg so that you can easily reach your foot. Sandwich your foot between the palms of your hands.

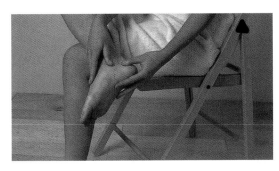

Working from your toes, massage towards your heel and ankle. Repeat several times.

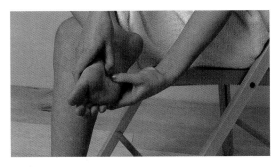

STEP 2 With your foot supported in your hands, fingers on top and thumbs underneath, work all over the sole of your foot with circular movements.

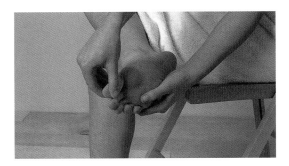

STEP 3 Support your foot in one hand and massage each toe with the thumb and fingers of the other hand. Start with your little toe and work along to your big toe.

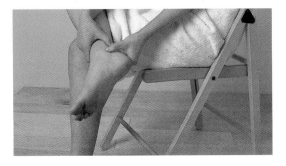

STEP 4 Massage all around your heel and ankle with your thumb using circular movements.

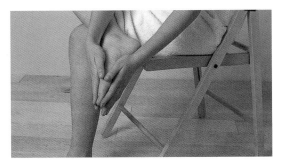

STEP 5 Finish by holding your foot between the palms of your hands. Press and hold, then gently lift your hands away.

skin Brushing

This is an excellent way of removing dead cells from the surface of the skin and for assisting the removal of toxins from the body. It helps to improve the lymphatic system and is particularly useful for the treatment of cellulitis.

The skin brushing is done on dry skin using a dry vegetable bristle brush. The brush must feel firm so it is important to start brushing gently and increase the pressure after a period of time.

For reasons of hygiene you should always use your own brush. The brush should be washed with warm soapy water once every two weeks.

The skin brushing should begin with the soles of the feet and work up the legs, front and back.

The abdomen can then be brushed in a circular direction. Then move on to the hands and up the arms. When brushing the chest and back, make sure that the strokes are always towards the heart. The back of the neck and the scalp can also be done, but avoid the face.

A few drops of a favourite essential oil can be added to the brush for added benefit.

As already mentioned this is an excellent way of improving circulation, stimulating the lymphatic system and removing toxins from the body and is excellent in the treatment of cellulite.

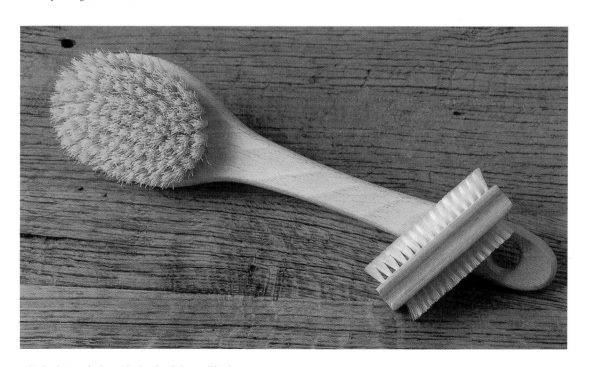

Skin brushing can be done with a long handled or small brush.

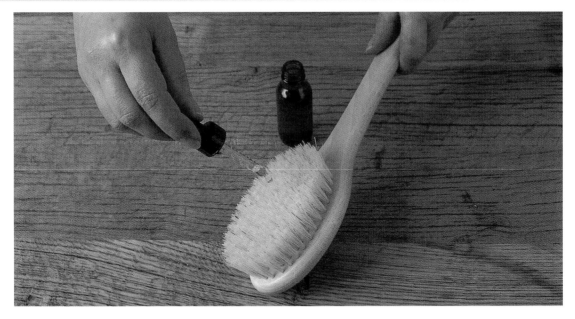

Add a few drops of your favourite essential oil to a dry brush.

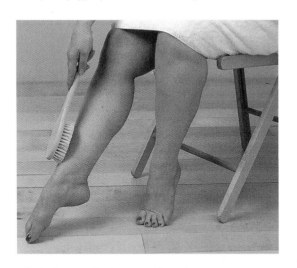

Skin brushing is excellent for improving the circulation.

IMPROVING THE LYMPHATIC SYSTEM

The lymphatic system can become sluggish which can affect the efficiency of the immune system, particularly during times of stress and illness.

The following advice will help to improve the lymphatic system.

1. Avoid mucous-forming foods. These type of foods increase congestion in the body. They include dairy products, red meats, refined white sugar and wheat products.

2. Eat lots of vegetables and fruit. These foods cleanse the lymph and blood due to the fact that they are rich in water.

3. Foot baths. Placing the feet in alternating bowls of hot and then cold water will improve the flow of blood and lymph. The bowls should be filled with enough water to reach ankle level. Tthe hot bath should be as hot as you can stand and the cold one equally cold. Place the feet in the hot water for three minutes and then into the cold water for one minute. Repeat about threetimes on a daily basis.

As well as correct diet, being able to breathe well and relax easily will be beneficial for you and those you massage. The breathing and relaxation exercises in the following chapters are based on Yoga techniques.

CORRECT BREATHING

Breathing is one of the most important functions of the body and all other functions depend on it. It therefore follows that incorrect breathing can impair the correct working of the body. Circulation can become sluggish causing fatigue, toxins can build up in the system and the digestive system can also be impaired. Shallow breathing does not give the body adequate energy which leaves people exhausted and more prone to stress.

Benefits which can be derived from the following breathing techniques are improved circulation, reduced tension, healthier body, increased oxygen supply to all body cells and extra vitality.

There are three distinct types of breathing:

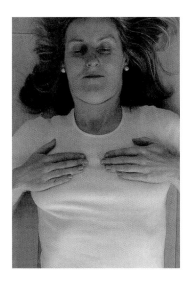 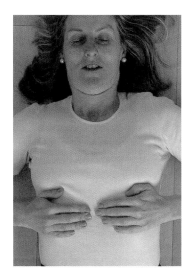 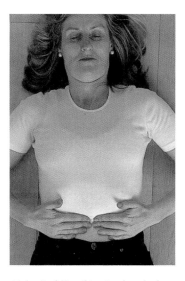

Clavicular Breathing is the most shallow type, where breath is introduced into the top of the lungs by the raising of the shoulder girdle, while the abdomen is contracted during inhalation. This type of breathing is natural to women.

Intercostal or Thoracic Breathing is done with the rib muscles expanding the rib cage. This takes a considerable amount of effort.

Abdominal Breathing is when the base of the lungs fill with air, aided by the lowering of the diaphragm. Men use this method automatically.

BREATHING TECHNIQUES

Important advice: although the following breathing exercises are very beneficial, if the person is suffering from heart or lung conditions they must check with their medical practitioner before attempting them.

COMPLETE BREATH

BENEFITS

This breathing method helps to energise the body and calm the mind. It is helpful in dealing with sleep problems and can be a useful boost in the middle of the day for people with demanding work schedules.

It is best to begin practising the Complete Breath lying on your back on the ground with your knees bent. In this way you can feel what is happening to your ribs and diaphragm when you breathe. When the technique is fully understood it can be practised sitting or standing.

1. Inhale into your abdomen by extending your abdominal muscles as far as is comfortable, allowing your diaphragm to move down.
2. Expand your rib cage so that your chest swells.
3. Raise your collar bones as far as possible without hunching your shoulders.

The Complete Breath cycle can be repeated several times, but four cycles are probably sufficient to begin with, building up over a period of time to around 20 cycles. Care must be taken to avoid hyperventilation.

COMPLETE BREATH

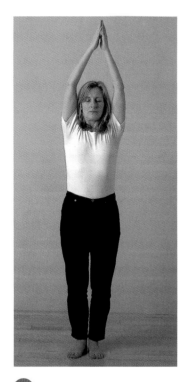

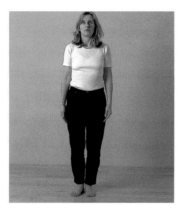

Stand erect with arms down by your side. Inhale steadily by extending your abdomen. At the same time begin to raise your arms sideways and upwards.

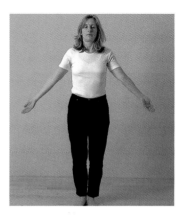

Continue inhaling, expanding the chest and pushing out the lower ribs. At the same time continue to raise your arms above your head.

The inhalation should continue until the both lungs are filled and your arms are fully extended above your head, palms touching.

Having fully inhaled, retain the breath for a few seconds, keeping your arms extended above your head.

Exhalation should be done slowly should incorporate the downward movement of your arms so that, when the breath is fully exhaled, your arms have returned to your sides.

ALTERNATE NOSTRIL BREATHING

BENEFITS

This breathing technique is useful for cleansing the sinuses and nasal passages. It helps calm the mind by balancing the nervous system.

Sit in an upright, comfortable position with your eyes closed. Thoroughly exhale out of both nostrils.

Press your left thumb along the left side of your nose into the inside corner of your eye socket. Your other fingers should extend horizontally across your face. (1)

Inhale slowly through the right nostril, and when fully inhaled block your right nostril with your fingers.(2)

Retain the breath for a few seconds. Release your thumb and exhale slowly out of your right nostril, continuing to block other nostril with your fingers. (3) Repeat this sequence a few times.

Then using your other hand, press your right thumb along the right side of your nose into the inside corner of your eye socket, with your other fingers extended across your face. Inhale through your left nostril.

Block both nostrils and retain the breath for a few seconds. Release thumb and exhale through your right nostril.Repeat this a few times.

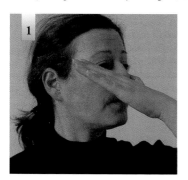 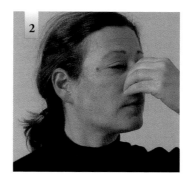 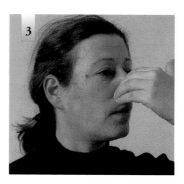

RELAXATION

Having studied various breathing techniques you should now look at some relaxation techniques.

Relaxation is simply an absence of tension or tightness. Although some tension is natural during physical exercise, we tend to suffer from constant tension, which causes unnecessary fatigue.

Breathing is also very important in connection with relaxation. The diaphragm relaxes during exhalation and when we let go of the diaphragm we let go of tension generally, so that when trying to relax we should relax a little more each time we exhale.

There are various positions that can be adopted for relaxation:

The Corpse position, or Savasan, is probably the most important position of all. It is performed lying on the back. The arms should be on the ground at about a 45° angle from the body, with palms facing upward and fingers slightly curled. The feet should be at least two feet apart with toes facing outwards.

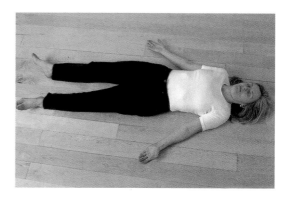

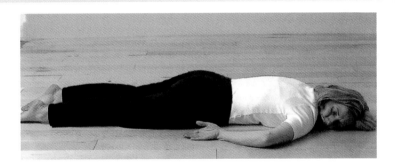

Your eyes should be closed and your face relaxed. The Prone position is practised lying face down on the floor. Your head should be turned so that one cheek is resting on the floor. Your hands should be by your sides with palms facing up. Your heels should be apart and toes pointing towards each other. Your eyes should be closed.

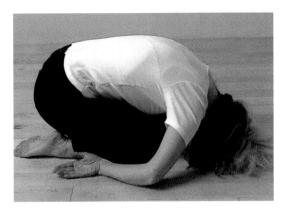

The Kneeling position is also known as the Pose of the Child. Kneel on the floor with knees together and toes pointing to the rear so that the tops of your toes are in contact with the floor. Arms should be down by your sides, and palms facing backwards. Slowly bend forward and lower your head until the highest part of your forehead rests on the floor in front of your knees. Lower your buttocks in the direction of your heels. At the same time bring your arms gently back, palms up, so they rest on the floor beside your body, hands beside the feet. Relax with your chest against your knees. Round your shoulders, close your eyes and hold this position for as long as it feels comfortable. Breathe normally.

The Standing position. Take up a comfortable standing position with your shoulders rounded forward so that your arms hang loosely in front of your body. Keeping your back erect but not stiff, relax your neck muscles and allow your head to hang forward so that your chin is resting on your upper chest. Again your eyes should be closed and the breathing normal.

RELAXATION TECHNIQUES

1 DEEP RELAXATION

Lie in the Savasan position as previously described. If you do not feel comfortable with the back of your head resting on the floor, a folded towel or small cushion can be placed under your neck and the small of your back. If you suffer from lower back pain it may help to lie with knees bent, then slowly lower your legs to the ground, easing the back into the floor.

Concentrate on relaxing the body muscle by muscle. Start at your feet, firstly each toe in turn, then move to your ankles, legs, knees and hips. Relax first one side of your body then the other. Now move on to relax your abdomen, waist, back and spine and your chest and ribs.

Relax your arms, starting with your fingers then move on to your hands, wrists, arms and shoulders. Again relax one side first, then the other. Then relax the back of your neck.

Move to the front of your neck and swallow to release any tension in your throat. Then relax your lower jaw and face. Try to smooth out any frown lines and close your eyelids very gently.

RELAX YOUR SCALP.

At first you may find this somewhat difficult and it may help to tense each muscle before relaxing it, so you can then feel the difference between tense and relaxed muscles.

These breathing and relaxation techniques combined with Aromatherapy and a sensible eating plan will help to improve your health and vitality.

Index

Picture Credits:
Quarto Publishing: pp 2, 6, 14, 52, 53t,
54.
E.T. archive: pp 8, 9.
ACE Photo Agency: 12t, 59t.

All other pictures © Quantum Books
Ltd.

Many thanks to the models:
Natalie, Aimee, Maria, Paula and Sarah.